YOUNG MIND YOUNG BODY

Transformational Approach to Rejuvenating Youth and Vitality

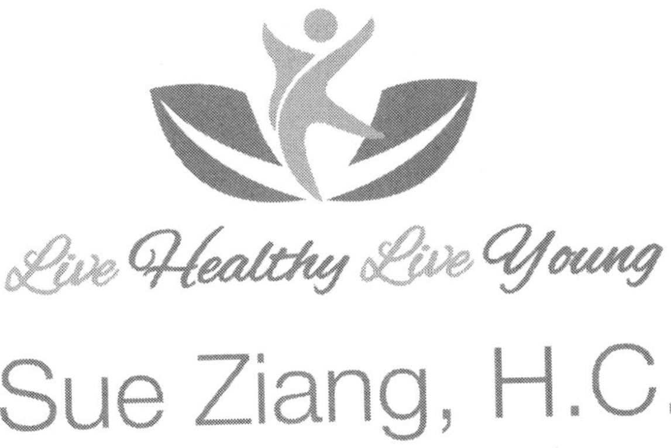

Sue Ziang, H.C.

YOUNG MIND YOUNG BODY
Transformational Approach to Rejuvenating Youth and Vitality

Published by:
Transformation Books
211 Pauline Drive #513
York, PA 17402
www.TransformationBooks.com

ISBN# 978-1-945252-06-8
Library of Congress Control No: 2016945353

Cover Design by: Ranilo Cabo
Layout and typesetting by: Ranilo Cabo
Editor: Allison Saia
Proofreader: Gwen Hoffnagle
Author Photo by: Michael Pix
Artwork by: grandpa_designs
Book Midwife: Carrie Jareed

Printed in the United States of America

YOUNG MIND YOUNG BODY

Transformational Approach to Rejuvenating Youth and Vitality

Endorsements

Sue intertwines her rich personal experiences with her life's learning, bringing forth *Young Mind Young Body.* Ignite your own healing through personal awareness with Sue guiding you back toward vitality, inside and out. You too may experience "gratitude attacks" and regain your timeless youth no matter what the clock says.

~**Pauline Kehoe,** *Self-Awareness and Transformation Healer; Five Element Acupuncture, M.Ac, L.Ac, Chinese Herbal Medicine, Medical Qigong Practitioner; Human Design Analyst, Human Design Career Analysis Consultant and BG5 Business Group Analyst. www.paulinekehoe.com*

My own life's transformational journey has led me to see the wisdom and insight embodied in *Young Mind Young Body*. Subtle shifts in mindset, supporting choices in lifestyle and foods, do shape our mind and body. The choice all along is in our own hands, as Sue Ziang has emphasized again and again, in so many different ways. Allow Sue's soulful healing words to inspire you to take actions laid out in her common-sense approach on your transformational journey of reclaiming youth and vitality, living the life you so desire living.

~**Charles Johnson,** *Qigong Level Three Master and Coach, Founder and Executive Director of MedSyn® Mind.Body.Soul. – a nonprofit organization promoting synergistic and holistic healing modalities. https://medsyn.us*

Should you seek to go for a walk amongst the trees of a forest or park; or should you have been searching for a wise "someone" to guide you through these trees? Maybe, you just want to walk side-by-side with someone who knows what you've been "going through." Then again, you may just want to listen-and-learn.

If so, then I invite you to casually "loop" your arm through the ready bend of Sue Ziang's willing arm who is, even now, welcoming you. Allow her to speak to your need. The rhythm of her words will reverberate the yearning of your heartbeat for a healthier life experience. Her enthusiastic and supportive guidance are yours for the day, any day.

This is her first English-language contribution dedicated to the simplicity of well-being and acquiring balance. The words she has proffered herewith will motivate deep-dwelling emotetions; the suggestions will woo you. Any reader will find this a surprisingly romantic book! Be willing to be its match!

~In truth, Gloria Garza, *C.N.H.P.; C.N.; C.I.; Inca Medicine Woman; Shaman*

I share a unique professional and personal relationship with Sue Ziang, proving that you can mix business and pleasure! Sue is truly an evolution in mind and body. Knowing Sue is knowing that growing up is not growing old. As she transparently shares her story, she exposes the road to gain and retain health, happiness, and abundance in all areas of life, while simplifying the process for easy digestion and personal integration. We are all in this life together, growing as we are going; the more you know, the more you grow. In her writing, Sue unfolds the map, intuitively becoming your compass, navigating the journey to optimal health. *Young Mind Young Body* speaks to all audiences with passion present on each page as well as knowledge and wisdom for every age! I am inspired and humbled to be on this path with her!

~Lauren Ranes | *AADP Health Advocate* | *Lifestyle Specialist*
Tenacious Wellness | *tenaciouswellness.com*
Tenacious Exploration | *tenaciousexploration.com*
lauren@tenaciouswellness.com | *330-354-5826*

Acknowledgments

Whoa! Where do I start? When my whole life turns into blessings wrapped in various outer wrapping papers, it is simply impossible to acknowledge everything and everyone that has sent me to the path leading my destined life. I will start with the basics that have helped me with the finished manuscript of *Young Mind Young Body*.

This book was written itself in life, right from my roots of growing up in China. On my healing journey home, I had this desire to put the book on paper. It was an idea for a while until I signed on with Christine Kloser's Get Your Book Done program. Finally, I started the downloading process of allowing the book to flow into different containers on pages, one bit at a time, in about two to three years' time. With the final push with my birthing team through Transformation Books, I am about ready to hold my baby in my arms and present it to the world in healing more lives, the same way it has healed me. Thank you, Tami, for signing me on with the publication package! Thank you, Carrie, for your mid-wifely patience, caring, and experience! Thank you, Allison, for gracing *Young Mind Young Body* with your editing expertise and endless laboring of love. Thank you, Gwen, for more editing and the final proofreading; your attention to details, your professionalism, your talents, and your passion for what you do have made *Young Mind Young Body* the best book it can be. I also want to extend my appreciation to Michele for making sure all the credits were properly secured and referenced. The book has become the way it is supposed to be because of you.

My friend Gloria Ganza comes to my mind. Gloria is a holistic health practitioner, an Inca Medicine Woman and Shaman. She and I met through the local GMO meetings I organized. Since then we have enjoyed each other's company in countless soulful chats over teas and easy friendship. Gloria always says that her friends come to her either because she can assist them or they need her companionship. I am the beneficiary on both accounts, her assistance and her companionship. One day out of the blue, she called me because she had this knowing that I needed her. As usual, we started talking, and naturally I told her about the book that was coming through me. Gloria said, "Now I know why I called you! I am supposed to edit your book. Here we go." She became the first path editor of *Young Mind Young Body*. She has poured her heart and soul, her language and writing skills, her expertise in holistic healing, as well as her outlook on life into the book. I honestly don't know what to say here except I am allowing the expansiveness of love and gratitude to roam free in me.

In the process of downloading the book, the universe sent many teachers to me in the spiritual realm. I was still sort of "seeking" in the phase of transporting the book onto pages. Gradually I have come to the realization that home was there waiting with open arms all along, whenever I was ready. The sensation of being home vibration residing in loving, unified oneness simply renders me speechless. What is there to talk about when all there is is stillness and nothingness? What is there to seek when we are singing to the beats of our heart song, immersing in source? Thank you, Bruce Adams! Thank you, Jim YOUNG! Thank you, Pete Heaton!

I am full of gratitude when I think of my peer coach, Lauren Rains. We have shared so many ups and downs, lows and highs, in our emotional and personal growth, and come to see the truth of ourselves through the mirroring. Nancy Baker, I am so very thankful for the airline trips and the drives we shared back and forth to training seminars invested in living our dreams, and the many nights in our shared hotel rooms coaching each other on the blockages and the steps. We have been on it non-stop, even in the middle of the nights when those *aha!* moments dawn. Thank you for your attentive ears and suggestions, and being present as a bouncing board when I was overwhelmed with the seemingly impossible task of editing! Thank you for sharing this unmapped journey with me!

To the man I married in the year 1996 due to my perceived insecurities and inadequacy, I am most grateful to you. Even in the most painful moment in your life, facing the divorce I imposed on you, you offered your time, your largeness, and your genuine support in reviewing *Young Mind Young Body*. I was moved to tears when you commented that my book is a piece of art, you couldn't put it down until you were done reading it, and that your only request was to have the first signed copy. All I can say at this moment is that "I have asked you to be that which you are so that I can be that which I am" in our soul contract, as Kayte Anna puts it eloquently in her book *Conscious Construction of the Soul*. I am so very grateful for the role you have agreed to play in the life we share together and in which we have raised a beautiful, kind, and intelligent soul who has agreed to be our daughter.

I can feel my face spreading into a content smile when the image of my precious daughter shows up in my mind's eye. Awww, Doll! You made me a mother, a role I thought I had lost the privilege to play, at the age of forty. You have been my rock, my teacher, my charge, my little girlfriend, and my mirror. I love you to the moon and back, countless times over. My life has forever changed with you in it. Thank you, Princess, for the many supports you have offered me in the process of bringing this book out of me. Thank you for challenging me! Thank you for being you so that I can be the mother I am supposed to be to support the person you are meant to be. Heck, you are part of the book and a partner on this path.

Now my attention turns to many friends and family who have asked to be the first ones to have a signed copy of *Young Mind Young Body*. The images of you come immediately to me: Lauren, Trent, Sean, Harry, Mara, Pamela, Mary, Mary, and Wayne, to name a few. And the countless many who have expressed the desire to buy the book, even multiples for friends as gifts, and the many store owners who are willing to sell *Young Mind Young Body* in the most prominent counter space of their store.

I am truly grateful to my coaching clients. YOU have taught me so much! Thank you for allowing me the privilege to be part of your journey in claiming your health and youthful vitality. You offered me the opportunity to experience firsthand what a blissful sensation it is to do the things I am called to do in this lifetime and be paid to do it. You have validated the notion that our dreams can support us in living the life we are destined to live when we apply and show up for ourselves, day in and day out, as a way of life.

I simply can't stop writing until I have acknowledged all of you, my readers, for purchasing *Young Mind Young Body,* supporting me supporting you. You are the reason this book is in print. Thank you with all my being!

This does not feel complete without acknowledging my first book client, Charles Johnson, Founder and Executive Director of MedSyn® Mind.Body.Soul. You entrusted to me your book tentatively titled *Mor.Fit – Magnificent Omnipotent Reality.Find in Time: Effective Ways to Transform Mundane Life to Blissful Living*. When you expressed your intention to hire me as a ghostwriter and collaborator on the book of your life, I was in the last phase of editing *Young Mind Young Body*, before it was sent to the publisher for review. Your unspoken endorsement, witnessed by your investment in yourself and in my ability as an author, has spoken volumes. Your ongoing unwavering trust in me in bringing forth the book that has been written through your actions, embracing adversaries and savoring living in the present moment in rare form, has infused a large dose of inspiration into my book-downloading process. I am so amazed by the way life evolves when we walk on the path we are supposed to be on, and how the universe conspires to send us the people we need to continue to live the life we are meant to live. It is meant that I am supposed to be awakened to the healing power of qigong through your book and your teachings. Your book is witnessing my further evolution after *Young Mind Young Body* and it will change countless lives just as it is witnessing the transformation of your life from severe depression to waking up every day feeling grateful and blissful. Thank you for showing up to yourself with weekly writings and constant insights. Thank you for allowing me the privilege of bringing forth a wonderful transformation book! Thank you for offering me the opportunity to learn and dive deep into medical qigong – the traditional Chinese healing art that is my natural inheritance! Thank you for the experience of doing the things I love doing until my last breath and being paid for doing them.

Last but not least, I want to thank myself for waking up to the truth of that which I am, showing up for myself day in and day out, getting this book out there, and spreading my rippling effect. I love you unconditionally! There is no shame, no apologies, no guilt in anything you have set out to do in the fourth chapter of your life. You are what you are, and I celebrate you for what you are. Thank you for finally having the wisdom and strength to be you! The universe would definitely lack your special imprint should you not have shown up as the authentic you, with your distinctive voice.

Yours in love and youthful vitality,
Sue Ziang, H.C.
Board Certified Holistic Health Practitioner
YOUNG MIND YOUNG BODY Health Coach
Certified Medical/Primordial Qigong Teacher
www.sueziang.com
www.youngmindyoungbody.com

Dedication

Dedicated to the men and women who are tired of being tired and want to claim lost youth and vitality so they can live the life they are born to live.

You want so much more out of life, yet you don't have the energy to go after that unfulfilled dream that renders you restless and unsatisfied. You find yourself harboring wishful thoughts: "How I wish I could live that way" or "If only I could live that life." YES! You can! The key has been in your hands all along. You have everything you ever need to have the robust, youthful health you want and to live the life you dream of living. Let's get started, shall we?

Table of Contents

Introduction

I grew up in China, in a time and place where life was simple and straightforward. Life was pretty much about following the ebbs and flows of nature, the cycles of the four seasons, and the rising and falling of the sun. It centered around working the land and basic sustaining, from planting, fertilizing, watering, working the soil, tending the crops, weeding, and harvesting to cooking, making clothes, and picking medicinal herbs from the field. During off-peak seasons, it was helping neighbors build houses; the men pitched in with all the actual building while the women fed the men and the kids. Food was largely plant-based, harvested from the fields, bartered, or bought locally, without much alteration from its natural forms. Eggs and meat were novelties and holiday affairs. In my memory, people were normally busy, lean, naturally fit, relaxed, happy, and content, even though there were not much of the material accumulations we possess nowadays. Of course, there were worries about not having enough to eat, not having enough material wealth to attract wives for sons to marry, or not being able to find a good man for the grown girl in the household to be married to. It was all part of living, and people took it in stride. No one stressed themselves to the extent of developing heart attacks. There were no such things as obesity and diabetes. Being "fat" was associated with being wealthy and affluent.

In January of 1993, I came to America to pursue my MBA and my long-cherished American dream. I pushed myself extremely hard, not knowing exactly what it was I really wanted except that I wanted to be successful and be somebody, proving myself worthy and capable. Graduating with an average of 3.7 on a scale of 4.0, I devoted myself wholeheartedly to the pursuit of my American dream. I worked in corporate America, built my own business and became my own boss, invested in real estate, lived in bigger and better houses, and experienced the life of fast food in the fast lane. Gradually home cooking became a novelty. Self-care was not a concept in my awareness. And the good habit of reading had given way to sitting on the couch watching TV. I remember boasting to some friends that I could eat anything without adding an ounce of weight to my body. It just proved how little I knew.

Suddenly it came to my attention that I was getting heavier and bigger. I remember hearing some people commenting that "The Americans are all rich like that, big and fat" when I was visiting my relatives in China. Even my daughter's dad was subtly hinting I was heavy by saying that the Chinese didn't do well on a standard American diet (the SAD diet). I had not been feeling well. Deep down I felt empty, tired, old, and ugly. Then, in 2003, I was diagnosed with high cholesterol and gestational diabetes when pregnant with my daughter. For a long time I was not able to bring myself to look in the mirror. The once youthful and vibrant face had worry, anger, fatigue, and age written all over it. There was this fog, which later on I learned from my readings was brain fog, clogging me from thinking clearly. Wear and tear had really done a number on me. I found myself constantly questioning the meaning of life: *Is this all there is to life? Could there be anything more to life? What is the point of living if all I am doing is driving myself to the bone to just pay bills for things that somehow don't even seem to matter?*

During the thickness of it all, my daughter was a toddler. I looked at her often, knowing that she was my heart and soul and that I should be able to love her to pieces, but I could not feel the love in my heart or the energy in my mind and body to fully participate in her life and give her the childhood she rightfully deserved. I was pretty much an empty shell, filled with anger and stress, barely coping with life's never-ending demands of running a business, cleaning the house, feeding the family, doing laundry, and constantly worrying about money. I was ready to jump the gun at any given moment, yelling and screaming. Talk about struggling with life, I was a walking billboard of that!

Occasionally the old dream of being something much more still surfaced. How I wished I had a magic wand to return to the youthful version of me again, full of hope and positive vibes, both in mind and body. The truth was that besides dealing with life's daily demands, I had nothing left for anything else, let alone dreams and wishes.

One day I heard a celebrity talking on the radio about surviving her cancer by choosing alternative treatments. She talked about her doctor telling her to put her affairs in order after she had refused chemotherapy treatment, and she lived to tell her story ten years later. Something clicked inside of me. My inborn sense kicked in, telling me there was something there. So I started my research, pretty much going through the self-help, nutrition, and food shelves at the local library, reading as much as I could get my hands on. In the process, my weight gradually came down, from close to 160 lbs. to about 115 lbs.

Over the years my natural ideal healthy body weight has found me, which is somewhere around 120 lbs. Not only have I easily kept the lost weight off, but I have also become healthier and more energetic. My brain fog has cleared up. Slowly clear thinking and sharper brain capacity came to me, assisting me in soaking up the nutrition and medical knowledge I was hungry for to increase my energy level. For a while I still struggled with the meaning of my life and thought it was probably too late to really live the life of my dream, but I started to have a glimpse of what the general direction should be: live healthy. At that point in my life, after tasting the wonders of feeling energetic and being able to think without the brain fog, I knew there was a better way of living and that life did not need to be always tiring and boring.

I never wanted to go back there again – feeling tired, fatigued, hopeless, depressed, and bitter. No way was I going to revert back to the way things had been! I knew I was on the path to something promising, so I was driven and propelled to quench the thirst for truth. One day when I was flipping through the books on the bookshelves in the library, I stumbled onto Deepak Chopra's book, *Ageless Body, Timeless Mind*. I was hooked, realizing that I could do anything I wanted to do in this lifetime, that my chronological age and the prison of self-imposed limiting beliefs should never be the walls between me and the life I longed to have. My reality was what I made it to be; what I perceived it to be.

As a natural extension of my research and the understanding of my unlimited potential as a being, I enrolled in the Health Coaching Training Program with the Institute for Integrative Nutrition (IIN), the largest online nutrition school in the world. I was afire to help people who were like I used to be, who wanted so much more out of life yet were too tired and fatigued to do anything besides fulfilling daily responsibilities. I wanted the whole world to know what I knew: how to live happy and healthy with youthful vigor and vitality and be the liveliest version of that which they were. Now I am an American Association of Drugless Practitioners (AADP) board certified holistic health practitioner and an IIN certified health coach. I have been assisting in transforming the lives of my coaching clients and those who are in my tribe through coaching, speaking, yoga, qigong and meditation teachings, social media postings, and spontaneous conversations with strangers. In the meantime, my life has been taking on newer heights. Just when I thought I knew enough, more awareness dawned on me. I am so very grateful that I have been experiencing constant gratitude attacks. My personal life and my professional life are together as one, merged in me, with me, like me, and through me, and delivering the message of rejuvenating youth and vitality. I am living the life I am meant to live.

While I am passionate in supporting stressed-out, worn-out entrepreneurs who are sick of being tired and ready to rekindle lost youth and vitality and prosper in all areas of life, the principles in *Young Mind Young Body* can benefit anyone who is ready to claim the life they are meant to live, rise above their circumstance, and assert their magnificence.

Once the core consciousness or soul is engaged, it is a rather simple way of living. All too often people who want more out of life, the free entrepreneurs at heart, are unconsciously driven to seek life's meaning and purpose. In the process, they are burdened by loads of stresses, chasing after superficial things. Their life force of vigor is severally depleted. Their body, face, mind, and heart show aging. This inner state of being can be reflected in outward bodily symptoms such as body weight. Instead of identifying the real cause of the weight gain, we go directly to the symptoms, looking for magic pills, chasing diet after diet, and going after shortcuts and prescription medicine. We go against our nature as beings who thrive on living in alignment with our environment, fighting battles by swimming upstream instead of downward sailing by savoring and living; that's to say if we are even paying any attention to our self-care at all. Many of us are forced to pay attention by a diagnosis of a serious or terminal disease that seems to draw a line in our life separating before and after.

What we don't realize is that it takes years of mindless living, from every thought we think, every emotion we feel, every response we respond to, everything we do or do not do, and every choice we make, to every bite of food we ingest, to get us where we are. The sudden onset of a heart attack, the accumulation of unhealthy body weight, the sluggish sugar metabolism, the clogging up of the brain, and the aged, worry-written face beat up the body; it doesn't just happen overnight. How we live our life, how we digest our food, and our life experiences matter. Mainstream media and commercial advertisements do not help, with the one-size-fits-all, no-need-to-do-anything-on-your-own, done-it-for-you approach that appeals to the mindset of instant gratification. In the end, it is a nation of sicker and sicker people, with over 50 percent obesity, over 30 percent diabetes, and stress-induced heart attack emergencies being the number one cause of death.

If you want so much more out of life, yet you are burdened with all sorts of baggage and too fatigued to go after your deepest dreams and desires, you are not alone. You worry a lot, your heart is not in your work or your job, you often think that if there were a choice you wouldn't be doing what you are currently doing. But you keep doing what you are doing because you have a family to support, bills to pay, appearances to keep up, and for heaven's sake, it is the life you know. You feel tired all the time, burned out, stressed out, thinking old, feeling old, acting old, looking old, and being old. It has been a long time since you had a good look at yourself in the mirror. Life is disappointing, full of struggles and uncertainties. You almost feel you want to be out of it. So naturally you start to amass stubborn belly fat and excessive weight. You have a hard time concentrating, thinking clearly, and acting with clarity. You think that you don't want to be like that, yet are hopeless for any change. Your doctor told you that you have high cholesterol or are showing signs of diabetes. You get angry and feel resentment building up, getting to a point where you cannot put up with this happy façade anymore. You want to yell, to scream, to cry about the injustice of life! Why me? Don't I deserve to be luckier than this? Where is this great destiny I somehow sensed deep inside of me? Where should I go from here?

I am here to say that there is a way, which is why I do what I do and why I wrote *Young Mind Young Body*. Life does not need to be a struggle. It is meant to be abundant and to be lived fully from your deepest wishes and wildest dreams. I have experienced firsthand how a subtle mindset and lifestyle shift and a change in food choices transform lives from daily struggling to effortless grace, from overwhelm to ease, from holding on to letting go, from fighting battles to following the ebbs and flows of life, from stagnation to creation, from fear to fearless, from hiding to freely expressing my uniqueness to the world, from overweight to a naturally healthy ideal body weight, from being angry with the world to being happy and at peace, from living to thriving, from ordinary to extraordinary, from mindlessness to mindfulness, from anxiety to peace of mind, from holding on to grudges to forgiving. In short, from thinking, feeling, looking, and being OLD to thinking, feeling, looking, and being YOUNG. I am growing young, body and mind, with my soul and heart fully engaged. I am feeling more alive, more vibrant than when I was in my twenties. Often I can't help but sing and skip a step while walking. I feel spring in my feet, music in my ear, and a song in my heart. I am living my dream and seeing it unfolding in the "here and now" awareness – that presence of mind that adds so much to daily life. (More about here-and-now awareness in chapter two.)

I have also witnessed lives transformed for my coaching clients. They come to me with seemingly different challenges on the surface, yet the same underlying cause: endless stress and worry from life's daily demands that stem from the disconnection from true self.

John is a business owner who had severe migraine headaches, a waistline that wouldn't shrink, and a temper that discouraged anyone from being near him. Yet now he is back to his ideal healthy body weight, his migraine headaches are practically gone, he is mellower, and he is in the process of writing more music and expanding his music business in recording and guitar teaching.

Wayne came to me with a taste of death in his mouth from sickness and sluggish immunity, wanting to be healthy and lose weight. About four months down the road, he was witnessing his stubborn body weight melt away. He was much calmer than before and was thriving at his job as a salesman with sales three times as high as the same time the previous year. He had received several promotions. In his email communications to me he wrote, "I am thankful to know you, and you have changed me more than you think. Thank you with all my heart."

My IIN community has endless stories of slowing down, curing, reversing, and healing. Almost everyone has a unique yet similar story to share. As a community, we share the vision of rippling our effect in healing the world at large while we live by what we preach: applying the healing power of supporting mindset, lifestyle, and food choices in our own self-love, self-care routine, and being the healthiest vision we can ever be.

The transformational approach presented in this book reflects the wisdom of ancient Eastern tradition and cutting-edge Western research. It is being practiced every day in all parts of the world where people are still enjoying the fruits of healthy, robust living and longevity, such as Okinawa, Japan; Montacute, England; Campodimele, Italy; Hunza, Pakistan; Loma Linda, USA; Nicoya, Costa Rica; Symi, Greece; Sardinia, Italy; and Bama District in GuangXi, China.

All of the above, and wellness-promoting teachings such as Chinese medicine, Ayurveda, and Greek medicine, have led me to the realization that a subtle shift in consciousness supporting mindset, lifestyle, and food choices is the key to building YOUNG MIND YOUNG BODY, slowing down or reversing early aging, and regaining a youthful appearance and vitality.

Sometimes I can't help but ponder that the approach to transformation has been made complicated. Being happy, healthy, and vibrant should be as natural as breathing. Then I reflect on my personal experience of getting lost in pursuits that were not in congruence with my core being and unconsciously following the social norm of viewing "having more" as the symbol of happiness and success. I realize that being healthy and young is so much more than just eating healthy, exercising, and following a good lifestyle. It needs the full engagement of the person as a whole – body, mind, heart, and soul – waking up from the inside; then being young and vibrant, mind and body, is just a natural by-product of living the optimal life we are meant to live, with meaning, abundance, peace, joy, and constant creation.

Young Mind Young Body is not about counting calories and learning the differences between fats and oils and how the body assimilates foods, even though these will be lightly touched on. It is about rejuvenating youth and vitality by applying self-love and self-care in all aspects of life. It is about starting from the source, cultivating and raising awareness, making supporting choices, and building everything into a daily bite-sized routine based on your uniqueness, preferences, ethnic background, schedules, priorities, likes and dislikes, circumstances, and the life you want to lead.

Rome was not built in a day, as the saying goes, and neither is building health and youth. Transformation is not about doing something major all at once. It is about taking baby steps and creating a daily routine that you enjoy, that fits your individuality, and that you can modify or make changes to as you see fit or circumstances require. Once you have the supporting habits in place, you can pretty much just follow the flow you have created for yourself and go on living your ideal life with ease and grace.

You have heard the fable of the Tortoise and the Hare. There is a deep implication in that story that reaching your goal or life purpose does not require you to be fast or to rush through things. It needs slow and steady effort, just like the tortoise. It is your youthful, vibrant health and true happiness flowing through your life that matter. Consistency and persistence are essential to creating a good house for your soul to experience the life you are here to experience.

This book is not meant for medical diagnosis; rather it is to wake you up to the truth that your health, your youth, your life, and your destiny are in your own hands. It is intended as a general guide to lead you towards building robust health and youth and using that rekindled youth and vitality as the launching pad to build and live the life of your dreams, the life you yearn to have. *Young Mind Young Body* is also intended to serve as a bridge to bring you to where I stand, and then you can step on my shoulders to continue your healing journey. After reading this book, if you feel in your heart that I am a good fit for you and you want more of me, I am honored to be your accountability partner, inspiring you to be the magnificent being you are and conspiring (co-inspiring) with you towards the life you dream of living.

I included many of the books I have read over the years in the References and Resources section in the back of the book. They have served me in gaining insight and perspectives in "building health building youth." I reference many leading experts in the wellness and healing industry and have asked for their permission to be included in my book or have informed them of my intent to do so. In order not to mislead you, I use the phrase "I have heard ... say" so that you know what I've written is my perception of what the person said. I am solely responsible for the content in case you don't quite decipher the expert's intent.

It is said that any thoughts you might be thinking, any impulses you might be experiencing, have all been said, done, or experienced before. In a true sense, we are all building onto one another with our own distinct imprints as our voices. The gratitude I feel at this moment towards all who have contributed to the collective consciousness pool is way beyond words. It simply renders me speechless. I can only immerse in the quietude of stillness in oneness to connect in love. Nonetheless, thank you from the bottom of my heart and the depth of my soul!

I asked my coaching clients for permission to mention them in the book. I can't even begin to say how grateful I am to them! I have learned so much from them! Thank you, my dear clients and friends, for allowing me the privilege to walk part of your healing journey.

Bear in mind that lasting, robust health requires a comprehensive transformational approach. Please understand that the underlying principle of total health transformation lies in interconnected and intricately linked overall mindful living.

If you feel I sometimes come on too strong, please know it is only because the love that came through me onto the pages was too strong. There are no judgments intended, only love. Where I repeat myself, it is simply the essence of my love and passion flowing onto the pages.

We all return to mother earth, merging with dust physically, and our essence stays in that unmanifested state of nothingness. We also share many other characteristics as human beings: we all eat, digest, think thoughts, sleep, and move. This is why certain lifestyles and food choices apply to everyone. We come here alone and will leave alone, in addition to many of the other biological and circumstantial differences and uniqueness. So there truly is no one-size-fits-all approach and application. Keep your mind and your heart open. Read with your whole being – body, mind, heart, and soul. Look for the resonance and apply what you feel is right in your gut. You know what is right for you deep down. Tune in to that inner knowing. Thank you for your openness.

Our essence has it all. Due to the transformational nature of my own personal journey, my intention to transform lives, and the nature of my coaching work, many of my experiential inner feelings and sensations show up in these pages, luring you to catch what I and many others on this transformational journey have been experiencing. The uplifting vibration from our truth as beings will speak with your dormant magnificence and resonate with your truth of love in oneness. Catch the fire! Shine your brilliance!

Chapter One

YOUNG MIND YOUNG BODY Building

1. Cultivate and Raise Your Awareness

Being aware is the first step in fundamentally transforming your life. It is said that the extent of your health is equal to the extent that you are aware of it. So many of us go through life blind, rushing without knowing, or avoiding knowing what is really going on. I lived a good part of my life like that; being born to a simple, healthy lifestyle, living through that life without consciously knowing the essence of it was the secret to vibrant health and the key to being naturally fit and slim without the need to be on any sort of diet. When we live in harmony with nature, life takes care of our bodies as a natural by-product.

My unawareness continued when I came to America, completely throwing myself into the pursuit of what I was conditioned to do: material accumulation and the expectation to retire from life by living on residual income. None of these are wrong in themselves; what was not right was to go after that life while not living in the here and now, at the cost of my health, going through life filled with constant stress, endless worries, and needless struggles. I ended up aged way before my time, mind, and body, carrying the symptoms of the modern-day American epidemic of an empty shell with the burden of weight, blood sugar dysfunction, and severe fatigue. The solution was there, but because of my limited beliefs and awareness, I struggled for many years, dating back to the early 2000s before my daughter was born. Once awareness dawned, it was like a light switch being turned on, gradually lighting up the darkness, illuminating everything in my daily life, just like a sunbeam penetrating the darkness.

Be aware of where you are in life, where you are as a person, how you feel about your life in general, and why you feel what you feel. Pay attention to your emotions in this process – what emotions are coming up and whether you catch yourself comparing your life to others. Give a rosy memory to the past and imagine a better future, but hate the way your life is at the current moment. Dig deep into your life, get in touch with your emotions, and start to understand yourself better.

You will also become aware that the state of your physical body is a reflection of your inner state of mind; your physical symptoms reflect your inner state of being, manifestations of your internal turmoil. For example, when you think old and feel old, you will gradually look old on the outside and your actions will reflect that of an older person. The saying "You are only as old as you think you are" applies here. Another example concerns obesity and diabetes; these reflect the accumulation of mind-induced stress and its effect on the body along with food and lifestyle choices. Lifestyle and food choices also contribute to heart disease, but the majority of heart attacks are stress-induced.

Modern science, a way of looking at the challenges we are facing today other than through the eyes of the heart, soul, and mystics, has proven without a shadow of a doubt that mind and body are intricately linked together. Upbeat feelings and a happy outlook towards life are associated with active left prefrontal cortex activities, while depression and negative takes on life, in general, activate the right side of the prefrontal cortex. Your thoughts and your emotions change the chemical messenger hormones in your brain. Happiness, or feeling good and peaceful, increases levels of serotonin, oxytocin, and dopamine, while on the other hand stress induces the hormone cortisol. These hormonal changes affect the brain and the rest of your body. Neuron receptors spread throughout your body, including to your heart, which is considered the neuro-cardio site; it not only pumps blood but also exercises emotional intelligence, such as feelings. Even more interesting, it is said your gut produces and stores about 95 percent of your happy hormone, serotonin, so gut feeling is nothing to be ignored or overlooked.

Your body is very fluid and very intelligent. It has built-in energy production, resource management, toxin removal, and a regeneration mechanism, with atomic particles flying around and information and energy as the life force. All of which are shaped by your thoughts, your awareness, your moods, your emotions, your actions, the food you take in, the fluids you drink, the movements you make, and the rest with which you honor your body. You shape and co-create the quality of your life – no more, no less.

When you do the right things to facilitate your body's smooth functioning and intelligence, it will do all the right things ensuring every part of your body is functioning at its optimal health and working order, where the cells communicate, interact, guard against viruses, and defend your body against alien attacks. Your body knows when you don't love yourself enough; don't exercise self-care; hide from feelings of pain, loss, self-shame, or self-guilt; or create any other self-imposed prison due to limiting beliefs.

Poor health can be caused by mindless living, including the coffee you might be drinking first thing in the morning, the missed breakfasts, the neglected lunches, packaged calorie-dense and nutrient-deficient snacks, overindulging at dinnertime, eating way too close to bedtime, and staying up late watching TV or surfing the internet when your body needs to rest the most to cleanse, restore, and repair itself and make new blood, or you need to simply connect with the inner you. The cycle continues against the very grain of living in alignment with nature. Your poor body can only borrow what it can to keep you functional with a minimal output of energy, trying to sustain life as long as possible until one day it can't do it anymore; it gets sick, with no reserves for repairs.

Hopefully you have awakened to the awareness early enough to aid your body in delaying or reversing the detrimental effects that have built up. It is what you do, think, see, feel, or are, day in and day out, that make the difference, and your body is the bearer of it all. Outside assistance, whether ancient or high-tech, can assist your body to the point of igniting its innate healing mechanism and performing its innate healing power. So it is imperative you make supporting choices in the here-and-now awareness to assist your body in giving you the quality of life you so deserve.

Sometimes feeling tired is a sign of your body's upward energy-building and healing, especially when you are on the healing journey and living mindfully. So are some cold symptoms, which are your body's way of releasing the internal dampness that builds up when the body is strong enough for some deep repairing.

On my own healing journey, just when I thought I had figured out all the things I needed to know to be at my optimal health and my natural body weight with constant highs, one summer I found myself feeling somewhat tired in the morning, even though I was calm, content, and happy with life in general and was at my ideal, natural, healthy weight and possessed clear thinking. A friend of mine, a Chinese medicine doctor by family tradition and by professional training, felt my pulse, telling me I was weak in yin, and yin-inflamed. This meant I had been tapping into my reserves of energy instead of making enough yang energy to meet the demands of my body. I couldn't quite make sense out of it, thinking that I had been doing all the right things and exercising self-care with my routines of early to bed, early to rise, morning meditation, doing yoga stretches while waiting for my hot water to be ready, eating a sustaining breakfast, choosing supporting perspectives on most occasions, and living life from the calm center. But I was eating hot and spicy foods, which further irritated the inflamed yin imbalance.

After much reading on Chinese medicine, I connected the dots to my puzzle: On my building-up trend, the quality and quantity of blood gained through mindful living had afforded me the boost of energy I felt at first; then the innate resource-management mechanism in my body decided to relocate some of the excess blood in my system to repair deep, internal damage caused by years of mindless living to further build up my immunity. At times I was stretching a bit too much, and tiredness showed up. Having a type-A personality, it's almost impossible not to push myself in this way. Tiredness can be more pronounced during the summer due to the body's adjusting to the hot weather and receiving less deep, restful sleep. Knowing this, I used every opportunity to aid my body in its repair work while maintaining my normal daily highs by staying away from the spicy foods that were inducing the inflamed yin state, and getting more restful sleep and restful awareness. I experience my highs again, where I am beyond content, calm, steady, and happy. A surge of energy pours through. I often feel spring in my step and find myself laughing for no reason and wearing a smile that comes from deep within.

Grow the awareness that as much as we are all the sum of our circumstances, you can rise above yours by being aware of your purpose for coming to this lifetime. Your soul chooses to experience certain experiences with your physical body as a vehicle to feel pain, joy, excitement, satisfaction, sexual desire, and so on, to come to the full awareness that you have it perfect as a being. Be aware of the truth that your desires, wishes, and dreams are here to guide you to stay on the course that your soul has set out for you.

Who do you think is observing or is aware of all that? It is the real you, your true essence, unchanging beneath the current of constant change and evolution. That is the other fact you will learn to be aware of once you grow accustomed to being aware of your inner and outer, the people around you, things around you, and many of the happenings in your life.

In the end, you will come to the awareness that the freedom of choice that comes from the totality of you as the being you are is the only thing that matters. I have struggled with this for many years, not quite understanding the reason for coming to America. It took going through all the hardships I created for myself to come to the understanding that happiness is as simple as a choice; so is a fulfilled life and my true destiny, which is all that has happened up to the here and now, with decisions coming from the deep place of being free. At the end of the day, you only have yourself to report to.

Being a spiritual being in your physical body, it takes constant, intense presence to reach the mastery of living. On one hand, your soul might not care about houses, money, wife or husband, lovers, kids, 401k, jobs, or cars, but your soul might need its physical house to be solid, sound, vibrant, and young in order to carry out its purpose. On the other hand, if the pursuit of the physical gets too far from the soul, then the zest, purpose, and vigor that come from the source drops or simply evaporates, which leaves your physical body to act from a disconnected place without a recharge or self-renewable energy. This then leads to a fatigued, worn-out, and aged state. You can pretty much trace back all modern-day disease to this disconnection with the source. If you just go all the way to a monk's life, with no accumulation of any worldly goods, and you feel the lack of these things, then that way of life is not your soul's purpose either, and you won't be able to experience certain experiences that come equipped with life's lows and highs. What I am getting at here is to be aware of how you are feeling. Any sense of loss, dissatisfaction, yearning, dreams, wishes, hopes, or aspirations is a sign from your soul telling you whether you are aligned or misaligned, guiding you as to where you need to be going. Once you come to this realization, your only guidance in life will be your gut intuition. Right and wrong, black and white, will gradually disappear from your perception. Everything has its place, and everything is about your perception and how it shapes or defines your reality the way you see it.

You can only perceive to the extent of where your awareness is. So raising awareness is essential. Be present to be aware of yourself, your thoughts, your emotions, and your responses to daily happenings. Be aware of what triggers your happiness response and what triggers you to feel anger and resentment; what excites and what bores you; why and how. Don't judge yourself by how you feel and how you react, just dig deep and develop this growing awareness. This insight will become wisdom, providing guidance on your healing journey and beyond.

Be aware that knowledge is power. Immerse yourself in a good, sustaining knowledge that you feel connected with by reading, observing, taking coaching sessions, and learning from life and people around you. Live with this knowledge; assimilate it in your own unique way that is your life and the way you live your life. Then this knowledge becomes wisdom, and a part of you, further assisting you on your healing journey with more insight and more awareness dawning on you in the here and now. It is an ongoing, lifelong journey. Go with it, taste it, enjoy it, and appreciate its many twists and turns instead of rushing through it for the sake of a mere destination. In the end, it is this journey of mindful living that counts, not that empty destination on the far horizon, once reached in haste, leaving you the feeling of being somewhat at a loss.

2. Shift Your Perception of Age and Aging

This is really big for me. The shift of perception towards age and aging has literally put a new life in front of me, enabling me to make choices I had never thought possible. Writing this book is just one of the physical testimonials of this new me. I constantly meet people who tell me that it is too late for them. So many younger ones in their late twenties and early thirties joke about being old, life being over for them, and it's too late to learn anything new. One time at a Chinese New Year's celebration, the program announcers constantly joked about how they envied the younger ones and how it was too late for them to learn new things. They couldn't help but feel the sadness and hopelessness of life, yet they looked awfully young to me. Coming from a culture where age plays a big factor in people's behavior, my take is that they probably said that to be liked and to fit into a certain mode of thinking, or maybe they were just following the patterns of their conditioned thinking or talking.

Let's take a look at definitions that relate to age and aging to crack the code. To define age, you and I look at time, age, chronological age, biological age, and the factors that influence aging.

What is time?

Einstein said put your hand on a hot stove for a minute and it seems like an hour; sit with a pretty girl for an hour and it seems like a minute. At a Chinese New Year's party a few years ago, we were invited to celebrate with the overseas Chinese students at Perdue Calumet. After enjoying the wonderful programs the students had performed, and socializing, we were all very hungry. The time we waited in line for the Chinese buffet felt very long, with aromas floating in the air teasing our senses and my then eleven-year-old daughter constantly reminding me how hungry she was. But in true time, it was only about ten minutes. We spent about one hour enjoying the feast, and I didn't hear anyone complaining about the time going slowly. It goes to say that time, while holding its position in the physical realm, is very much subject to interpretation based on one's circumstances, emotions, state of mind, and physical body.

Two Chinese sayings come to mind when it comes to the interpretation of time. One is "Time flies like a rocket," connoting the notion that when everything goes well, time just flies by. While another saying, "It felt like a year going through one day," pretty much sums up the agitated state when one is struggling or having a hard time or not feeling well emotionally or physically. Yes, you could say that there is real time, proved by your watch, your cell phone clock, or the clocks on the wall, clicking away and waiting for no one. But where do these time-clicking devices come from? They are inventions of humankind for referencing things. There is also a Chinese folk song, "My Family Lives on the Yellow Plateau," that says, "Wind blows, different time different seasons of the year, it is always my song, whether it is eight hundred years or ten thousand years," indicating the wisdom of timelessness. When I stare out of the window observing snowflakes flying and falling, all I see is eternity and timelessness. I don't see time written anywhere on this beautiful scene. Have you ever seen time flying by in nature? True, you see flowers bloom, leaves turn, fruits grow bigger, but that's just the natural sequence of things indicating changes in the physical realm where our bodies exist, which is probably why humankind invented time in the first place. Einstein also said that the only reason for time is so that everything doesn't happen at once.

In that quietness you sometimes feel when you close your eyes, where there are no thoughts, you hear the sound of stillness that is the essence of timelessness, the essence and true nature of all the beings. That is why you can feel its existence in rare moments when you are in the presence of ideal love, love that makes your hearts skip a beat, where you stare into each other's eyes yearning to join beyond the physical into infinity and eternity. Time simply stays still. It is also in this state that time ceases to wear and tear on you. In these moments you have escaped the metrics of time, its implications, and its aging effect on you. So the question is, how can you be in that timeless dimension more often, with longer duration, allowing your body to tap into that fountain of youth, or timeless quality?

Now that we have a grasp on the true concept of time, let's take a look at age. ***What exactly is age?*** Age by its official definition is the number of years a person has lived to the current point. Now we understand that time is made up to reference things so that events can play out in sequence. Since age builds upon time, this characteristic makes age very much up to interpretation, very fluid, very personal. It is not as concrete or solid as you and I have come to believe. It can be influenced by everything we do or don't do, by every thought, by every emotion, by the way we assimilate our life experiences, and by the way we live our lives. Most of us assign it too much power to determine what we should or shouldn't be doing.

There are two concepts of age: chronological age and biological age.

Chronological age is the number of our accumulated years based on the manmade calendar. In the old days, a stick was placed on a wall for one day, seven for a cycle of seven days, and more for a month and a year by observing the rotation of the sun and our relative position to it. Then there is the Western calendar system based on the rotation of the sun, and the Chinese lunar year calendar based on the rotation of the moon relative to the sun and to our home planet Earth. Throughout history, time and years have been created to facilitate the activities of farming. Time comes from nowhere, just like the timer on your cell phone. Manufacturers put it there based on generally accepted rules.

Over the years, people of different origins have agreed on certain ages for certain things, such as childhood years to play, study, and prepare for a life to be lived; late teens and early twenties to study in colleges and universities, preparing for a career for the balance of a person's life; then it is work, marriage, having kids, buying a house, and settling down, creating a certain pattern for this whole life. In your fifties and sixties, you are supposed to have accumulated enough and worked enough. Now you can think about taking yourself away from all this working, since that is what you have been doing ever since you shouldered a mortgage, kids, and your kids' education. Now it is your time for a break. If you need to keep working, either based on necessity or choice, you will be one of the odd birds. You will even feel that way yourself since you are conditioned to this way of life. You have seen your parents and people all around you doing it, and a whole industry for the retirement sector has been created just for that purpose. So now it is time for you to just kick back, relax, and enjoy the fruits of life.

But wait a minute; what if you don't want to retire? What if you feel like you have just started to grow up? What if you still feel young, alive, and vibrant, with passion inside, ready to set the whole world on fire? What if you want something more out of life? What if you feel a piece is missing, and you want to work at something until the moment you breathe out your last breath? Should your chronological age hold you back? Why should numbers in years in this world have any bearing on you or me or anyone else in this matter, as long as we are alive and kicking, feeling the energy of our twenties? I have decided I can feel the energy I felt in my twenties; I have been doing it and intend to live this way until the moment I am ready to drop my physical house that is my body. So can you!

As you can see already, chronological age does not determine how young or old you really are. All it says is that you have been here for a certain number of earth's rotations of the sun. Most of the time it is the limiting beliefs imprinted into our consciousness that hold us prisoner in our chronological age. Once you know the truth, you don't have to be influenced by that. No need to feel old and tired just because you are thirty, or forty, or fifty, or sixty, or seventy, or a hundred. There is always someone younger than you in chronological age. And there is always someone older than you – for most of us anyway. If by some miracle you and I are the oldest in chronological age, then we have done something very right. Congratulations! Then we can show the world how it can be done!

Think outside the box about chronological age dictating whether you should die, live, study, learn, or just take it easy. Study when your heart craves it. Start doing that thing you have always wanted to do if you feel called to it.

Biological age involves biomarkers of aging "that better predict functional capacity at a later age than chronological age. Stated another way, biomarkers of aging would give the true 'biological age,' which may be different from the chronological age" (Wikipedia). You probably have heard the saying "You are as old as your oldest organ." Biological age is your real age. Accumulation of years seems to have very little impact on some people's faces, bodies, and minds, as if the universe kisses the very ground they walk on. While for others, years and time seem to really do a number on them, with age showing up everywhere in their very being – in their thoughts, in their words, and in the way they react to the outside world.

I have a distribution business, and I was chatting with one of my suppliers once about aging and life in general. He commented that he could pretty much tell a person how they lived their life just by looking at their face: the worry lines, the wrinkles, the complexion, the texture, the color, and the emotions evident. He said he was always right. The medical field is also using biomarkers as a measure of real age. You might have heard your doctor say that you have the heart of a thirty-year-old when you are fifty in calendar years; on the other hand, I have heard so much about our ten-year-olds having the hearts of fifty-year-olds, the first generation that might be dying ahead of older generations if drastic lifestyle changes are not implemented.

What is aging?

Overall effects of aging include reduced immunity, loss of muscle strength, decline in memory and other aspects of cognition, loss of hair color, and loss of elasticity of the skin. The integrative biologist Dr. Joao Pedro De Magalhaes, in Senescence.info, defines it as "a progressive…deterioration of physiological function…or the intrinsic…age-related process of loss of viability and increase in vulnerability." More research turns up similar results describing the decline of bodily functions. Aging is not really defined as time or age; it's the bodily symptoms associated with them.

Being young starts with the mind. All it takes is for you to start understanding the truth, which is that your mind influences your body at the deepest level, and to learn to take action in tapping into that timeless essence. Your physical body can do all the right things, make all the right choices, coordinate all the right actions, with 100 trillion cells performing a hundred thousand functions at the same time – communicating, responding, supporting, backing up, defending one another, even sacrificing themselves – to protect your body. Your mind does the rest.

In quantum physics, everything invisible to the physical eye is a swirl of flying particles with no directions, no shapes, no time. When being observed, they attain an orderly pattern, which goes to say that attention influences things. That is the way the cosmos operates at its core. We are part of the cosmic being, driven by the same life force and operating in the same ways on the most basic level, even though our physical eyes can't see that dimension. It is very important that you understand this concept because the cells in your body listen in on your thoughts, interpret your emotions, and then coordinate a sequence of communications and actions through chemical messengers to manifest what's in your mind on the physical plane. So everything you do influences the way your body ages.

When you think young, you take action, do things with youthful vibrancy, and don't allow your chronological age to be the determining factor of your destiny. As long as you feel youth in your very being, it manifests in your body. Youth shows up on your face and vitality shows up in your being, while some of the accumulated wrinkles and signs of age start to disappear. The key lies in your perception of time, your interpretation of its meaning, and whether or not you give power over to society's definition of time to influence you.

This physical body of ours, our temporary house in this lifetime on the physical plane, is governed by physical laws. Seasons come and go; trees sprout in the spring, flower in the summer, bear fruit in the fall, and become dormant in the winter. They come back to green again when spring comes along. There are many factors affecting how we age. We cannot control some of the mysterious ones like the law of constant change in the physical realm, manifesting as the natural law of birth, growth, suppression, and decay. Animals might not realize they are getting old when the aging process takes place in their bodies; humans, on the other hand, are fully aware of this process, and we can stop, slow down, or reverse aging to the extent we use our awareness.

Aging is very individual, very fluid, and can be affected by the here-and-now choices we make. My focus in this book is the factors in regaining lost youth and vitality that are in our hands, from subtle shifts in consciousness to mindset, lifestyle, and food choices. I don't talk about the mysterious factors or natural order of things that we cannot control. These factors are out of our hands and we must trust that the universe will support us as the beings we are and that these factors work for our evolution. And they will if we collectively cultivate the right intention and raise our awareness.

But there is a whole lot we can do to stop, slow down, or reverse the detrimental effect aging has on us and rejuvenate youthful vitality, just by making good supporting choices in how we think, how we perceive things, how we assimilate our emotions and life experiences, how we go about our daily lives, and how, what, and when we eat to feed our bodies.

I am not talking about living beyond 100 years young, even though the prospect is very attractive. I am talking about rejuvenating youthful vitality – being able to think young, feel young, look young, and be young and vibrant again – especially if you are feeling old and worn out. What would your life be like if you could feel and look up to fifteen years younger? It is up to you, in your here-and-now decisions. Make a decision in this moment about how much younger you would like to be, then think, act, and behave from that age.

Many books have been written about this subject. Dr. Deepak Chopra included ten practical steps for reversing aging in his book *Grow Younger, Live Longer* that can be applied in a habit-forming process to help us reestablish a new *biostat,* which is the ideal biological age we want to be, up to about fifteen years younger than our age in clock time. Dr. Eric R. Braverman subtitled his book *Younger You* with *Unlock the Hidden Power of Your Brain to Look and Feel 15 Years Younger*. Bob Greene, author of the #1 *New York Times* bestseller *The Best Life Diet*, authored another book titled *20 Years Younger*. Dr. Mehmet C. Oz co-authored the book *You Staying Younger: The Owner's Manual for Extending Your Warranty* with Dr. Michael F. Roizen, and motivates his readers to incorporate vital habits into their daily lives so that staying young becomes a routine habit.

Starting today, look at the timers on your kitchen counter, your digital clocks, your cell phone, and your old-fashioned wall clocks with a new insight and supporting perspective. Remind yourself that humans manufactured all these devices and you bought them for the convenience of being in sync with everyone else around you. Can you imagine what chaos there would be without time reference – those missed appointments and dates – and no modern-day scheduling? So use time to that extent, no more and no less.

Time has nothing to do with aging. You can escape its hold on you, slow down the aging process, and maybe reverse the early signs and symptoms of aging.

Go to the woods for long weekends, where timelessness reveals its beauty and eternity and demonstrates its wisdom. It will impact you and instill in you that same beauty, eternity, and wisdom. Every time you experience timelessness, your body slows down or stops, reversing the aging process.

3. Building Youth Is Building Health

YOUNG MIND YOUNG BODY Defined

Youth is associated with robust health, both in mind and body. A youthful body is free of disease and is able to bounce back quickly once sick. So building *youth* is building *health,* in every sense. Reclaiming youth and vibrancy also means reversing many of the physical symptoms of disease and enjoying a life of enhanced well-being. Building youth and building health go hand in hand with fully engaging your soul, or core consciousness, and the emergence of your true self and your supporting mindset, lifestyle, and food choices.

We have all heard people talk about being too late, too old, too set, or too busy to do the things they want to do in life. Deep down they know these are excuses for not facing their true, powerful selves. These people skip over the surface of life and never experience the exhilaration that comes from expanding your comfort zone. Separating from the source and living from your ego can result in feeling burned out, fatigued, exhausted, tired, and beat. A young mind and young body begin with these concepts:

- You don't just grow old; you *become* old when you stop growing. As long as you live life with an open mind and heart by staying intensely present, you will be forever young. It's only when you stop growing that you start becoming old.

- Your physical body, the house of your soul, is a dynamic living organism. It is in a constant state of renewal and regeneration in which new cells grow, old cells die, and your body is totally new in about a year's time. A healthy lifestyle facilitates building new cells, improving digestive and lymphatic movement, and increasing quality of blood and therefore *qi* – vital energy, finally letting the truth of you come out as the person you are. This includes food intake, physical body movements that stretch muscles and flex bones, the way your body assimilates and digests food, the manner in which you "inhale" and process your life and emotional experiences, and all the other supporting choices you make in you're here-and-now awareness.

- Age is just a number, not a factor in determining your fate. It is simply the accumulation of years that you have been alive. The concept of a year was created to measure the evolution of cosmic beings. Various other measurements have been invented for such purposes such as seconds, minutes, hours, days, weeks, and months. In essence, time does not exist. It is all the particles swirling around with no direction, shape, or meaning until humans assign it a definition for the purpose of reference.

- It is never too late to follow your dreams and deepest desires. Life is about *experience experiencing experiences*. It has nothing to do with how old or young you are. It has everything to do with being content doing what you were born to be doing. It is about living your dreams, living fully and optimally, and tapping into your potential. Holding back, getting caught up in life's commotions, or getting deeply depressed or intolerant of your physical existence can only leave negative imprints in your subconscious. You will start over where you left off, somewhere down the road of your soul's journey, with similar circumstances and similar casts of characters. It truly pays to live life boldly in your physical body in the here and now.

- Your essence is so fluid that it can be wrapped around you to be what you want it to be, your wish being its command. At your core, it is the fluid, dark matter full of unlimited potential and possibility to be shaped and drafted to the way you wish things to be, like a white piece of paper in front of you waiting for you to draw the most beautiful or ugly picture you have in your mind.

- Challenges are blessings and opportunities in disguise. Embrace challenges instead of avoiding them. They are here to show you what you really are and lead you to the path of your true calling.

- Change is in your essential nature and is inevitable against the backdrop of non-changing stillness and quietness. It is the theme of life, from the cells deep in your body to everything around you – the seamless change of seasons, days into dusks into nights, rainy days, snowy days, and changing emotions. "No man can ever step into the same river twice," said the Greek philosopher Heraclitus. Change is what keeps you from being stale and old, and it keeps the fresh blood of creation going. It is the wisdom of unpredictability at work.

- Uncertainty is your certainty. You don't know what's going to happen in the long run or on a day-to-day basis, who is going to show up in your life, or what's going to happen to your financial well-being or your well-being in general. You are okay with knowing that uncertainty is the root of creation, expansion, living your unlimited potential, revealing the real you, and feeling the bliss of life. You only need to be present in the here and now and embrace uncertainty with open arms and an open heart, savor its flavors, and learn from the lessons showing up. Or simply interact with love and allow life to unfold.

- Abundance is your birthright. You look around and see everything in nature's abundant supply: running water, free air, fruits in the trees, bushes blooming, flowers thriving, beautiful sunshine, the endless harvest of foods, the love in the smile of a stranger, the kindness in a friendly hello, the beauty in a beautiful soul telling you how beautiful you are, the friendship in an afternoon chat with someone you can pour out your heart to, the tranquility in the moment of calm and peace with the sound of stillness wrapping you in safety, the fun and aliveness of life in a harmless flirt, and the compassion of a stranger standing next to you in a checkout line offering you the few dollars you are short of to get the last item you want. You have everything to sustain your life on planet Earth. You are and will be taken care of abundantly.

- When there are ups, there are downs. It is like so many other polar opposites: where there is north, there is south; there is yin, there is yang; there is happiness, there is sadness – opposite ends of the same spectrum. All is good. You can always lift yourself to where you feel the most peaceful and vibrate at love frequency. Once you have experienced this, you can always reach a higher plateau.

- It is a divine right to be able to make choices from that place of total freedom. It is also a divine responsibility. True freedom derives from deep within, where you align your outer self with your impulses, your true calling, and the purpose that is directed by your gut intuition. Your desires, your dreams, and your wishes are clues that your soul is directing you to be on course. Make wise choices to live the life you are destined to live.

- Your life is solely your responsibility; no one else is to blame for whatever is happening in your life. Take charge of your life, even when you accept true giving, help, and collaboration with gratitude. If you don't like what you see, even though you accept your now as is, view it as a lesson or a message with no blaming. Then implement change to where you want to be.

A young body is naturally fit, healthy, and free of everyday disease, with robust immunity. If disease does occur, it is able to experience shorter durations and less severity than an unfit body, and bounce back more quickly. It carries with it a glowing and youthful-looking face and it is full of energy and vibration, able to support living the life of your dreams. These are the benefits you will potentially reap by following the YOUNG MIND YOUNG BODY building system outlined in this book and breaking it down into bite-sized daily habits.

Building Up Robust Health and Youthful Vitality

The YOUNG MIND YOUNG BODY building principles are intended to help improve the stage of *secondary health.* Chinese medicine defines this as the stage of health between robust health in all areas of life, including enjoying high energy frequency; and the other extreme – the full physical and mental manifestation of illness in which one is completely exhausted, depleted, and fatigued. There are five stages, broken down by diseases and symptoms associated with blood volume in the body by using the concept of yin-yang, weakness and strength, according to *The User's Manual for Human Body (人体使用手册)* by Qing Zhong Wu (吴清忠). This book illustrates Chinese medicine from the perspective of modern-day information technology and resource management. The following description is what I have assimilated about the five stages from reading Mr. Wu's book, though it barely scratches the surface given the complexity of the Chinese medicine system.

- **Robust health**: Chinese medicine perceives yin-yang balance as the goal of perfect healing. People in this stage are perfectly balanced in all areas of life, lacking neither yin nor yang and neither too weak nor too overbearing in any one area. They have the characteristics of a well-balanced body: pink, rosy cheeks; a mild temper; happiness; radiance; and a healthful daily routine. People in this category have strong immunity and hardly ever get sick. Few people enjoy this stage of health given modern-day living. Most of those who do practice meditation, yoga, qigong, and other mind-body building routines with persistence and constancy.

- **Yang-stage weakness**: Blood volume and quality are not as good as those of a person in the robust health stage. Blood and *qi* are in decline. The level of immunity and the point at which disease breaks in get fairly close. Therefore the body is in a constant symptomatic state because it takes longer for it to get rid of viruses and other alien invaders. People in this stage might appear to be constantly sick with minor illnesses.

- **Yin-stage weakness**: Due to long-term stress, worries, and pushing the body too hard, it further declines in blood and *qi*. It is very common in today's society to burn the midnight oil, causing depleted energy reserves. The duration of this stage varies depending on the person's overall lifestyle. It can last twenty, thirty, even forty years until one day the person starts to feel sick, goes to the hospital, and is diagnosed as having cancer or heart disease. The interesting thing about this stage is that because the body is so weak and immunity is so impaired, viruses and alien invaders come right in without any resistance from the body. So there are no signs of resistance in the form of symptoms. Someone in this stage might think they are healthy since they are hardly ever sick, but the wear and tear is there in facial skin tone and body shape. The internal organs silently take the beating and are only able to perform necessary daily functions with no strength for repair and restoration.

- **Both yin and yang stage weakness**: Further decline continues to deplete the body to a point where all energy reserves have been used up. To maintain minimum output while sustaining life, the body starts to eat into its own tissues, organs, and muscles, heading towards constant fatigue and exhaustion.

- **Total exhaustion:** This occurs as the downward decline in blood volume and quality continues. At this stage, internal resources have been depleted to a point where the liver is constantly inflamed in its effort to produce energy and keep the body functioning. This causes an inability to sleep at night, further depleting the body and inflaming the liver. It is a ferocious cycle. Poor quality sleep and short duration of sleep impair the body to a point where digestion, assimilation, and absorption are hindered due to a blocked gall bladder and reduced secretion of digestive juice. Many serious life-threating, no-cure diseases such as various forms of cancer accompany this stage until death claims the physical body and releases the soul if nothing is done to halt or reverse the process.

The decline of blood and energy takes a long time and is different for every person. The rate of decline depends on many factors such as the starting state of health, the duration and quality of sleep as a child, eating habits, and general outlook on life.

Feeling old often accompanies physical decline. This is also when modern-day epidemics manifest in the physical body. Declining health is a sure path to full onset of disease, and once it develops, medical treatment can only ease the pain or control its further progression.

Building towards robust health can result in obvious improvements fairly quickly. One can feel better and rested in perhaps a month, achieve noticeable outward differences such as better skin tone in six months, and start to turn things around in a year or two. Accompanying this upward trend are the many internal repairs happening simultaneously. They are determined by the body's innate resource-management system, which intuitively knows what to do with more available blood in the body. It is sort of like running a business. When there is more and more income coming in, more will be spent on building up company strength and branding. At times you might feel fatigued, especially in the summer when blood is being directed to do some deep repairing. Symptoms that modern medicine calls disease can accompany this building-up trend. This is the body's way of releasing toxins that have accumulated and been trapped deep inside for years as it gains enough strength to do so. All too often drug treatments stop this natural bodily healing in its tracks by interfering with the body's healing mechanism. The ideal objective of any outside intervention should be to build up the body so it can activate its innate healing power, healing itself by itself.

Addressing declining stages of health with the comprehensive approach laid out in this book can prevent or delay many serious diseases such as heart disease (the number one killer in America) and cancer (the number two killer).The approach is low-tech and low-cost compared to the high-tech high cost of our current medical system. Many causes of disease can be erased through a shift in consciousness and through mindset, lifestyle, and food choices. It is said that 90 percent of our problems are due to our lifestyle and food choices. We live ourselves into this epidemic, so we can surely live ourselves out of it. This approach is simple, intuitive, straightforward, and easy to follow, yet life-changing. All you need is a willingness to take charge of your health, find what works for you, and modify it and keep at it for the balance of your life.

4. The Benefits of Applying YOUNG MIND YOUNG BODY Building Principles

Being healthy and vibrant is your birthright. By stripping off all your trappings and decorative layers and living from the source, you can live optimally; enjoy a vibrant, young mind and a vibrant, young body; go about life with ease and grace; and do what your heart is called to do. You might also experience the following perks as natural by-products of living in alignment with your deepest desires. Who wouldn't want this, I often wonder?

- **Slowing down, stopping, or even reversing your aging process:** So much age is added to your face and body by struggling through life and worrying about money, kids, and everything else. You come to look old way before your time. It slowly but surely depletes your body's reserves, drains blood quality and quantity, and reduces vital energy or *qi* so that a sufficient amount cannot be transported to various parts of the body, including the brain. Your immune system cannot function at its best in guarding against alien invaders. This, in turn, causes deterioration in bodily functions, making you look and feel older, with signs of age-related diseases.

But you don't have to live that way. Living the transformational approach to your daily life – treating yourself as the whole that you are in body, mind, heart, and soul – allows you to slow down the roller coaster of aging, stop its rapid progress, and even reverse the aging process and regain lost vitality. The key is in your own hands. You might be thinking that genes play some role in this, or that aging can't really be halted or reversed, and yes, genes do play a role – but a very small one. You can't change your inherited genes, but you can change *expression* of those genes by turning some on and some off through constant attention to your health and well-being. This has been proven beyond a shadow of a doubt. You don't need to take anyone's word for it; just see it for yourself, and you will be rewarded with renewed youth and vitality. It is a known fact that many so-called aging symptoms can be reversed or eliminated with a subtle shift in consciousness and supporting mindset, lifestyle, and food choices. There are more and more vibrant, youthful-looking people in their forties, fifties, and sixties living their passions and dreams than ever. This can be you, too. Though there is no known way to stop aging altogether, there is growing evidence that many things can be done to suspend or reverse that process for some time.

- **Starting to feel young, think young, look young, act young, and be young:** Being young can be felt as a feeling, a thought, a look, an action, or a reflection of your core being. You simply come alive and do that something you have been dreaming of doing since childhood but were too tired to even try. You constantly hear comments about how young you look or that you haven't aged a bit. Younger folks flirt with you. People with the same energy are drawn to that youthful, robust vibration – that fire, that spark, that life deep within. You are on fire, in your element, in your core, being the most authentic you.

- **Being more vibrant and having enough organic energy to go through the whole day without the afternoon energy crash:** You don't need a morning cup of coffee or any other caffeinated drinks to wake you up by stimulating the production of adrenaline – the fight-or-flight hormone that gets you going but depletes your energy reserves. The daily habits you create for building health and building youth bring your body to its organic best with everything coming from your body's innate intelligence, keeping you at your peak performance level. This organic energy carries you from the time you get up until your natural bedtime. Then you are ready for rejuvenating sleep with your body temperature normal and your liver functioning optimally. This enables you to sleep deeply and peacefully and get up feeling rested, restored, refreshed, and rejuvenated, ready for a day of excitement.

Most people who work during the day feel tired around three in the afternoon and need to eat something quick to get through the rest of their day. This is the body's craving for more energy. Eating sugary snacks is the easiest way to provide the body with energy in the form of glucose, so most people just grab those, or coffee, providing a lift. This slides you further into the rabbit hole. If you have taken care of your body by applying self-care and self-love in your daily routine, chances are you won't need that stuff to begin with; the "crash" will be a thing of the past. Even when you feel some tiredness, a power nap or meditation takes care of it. You can simply sit in your chair or in your car, close your eyes, drop into the space in between thoughts, and feel invigorated and rejuvenated. Any short period of time will do – maybe five minutes, maybe ten, or a half hour. It beats coffee and sugary drinks and snacks any day.

- **Watching the challenging weight melt away just by living the life you love to live:** No need to try diet after diet, challenge your will to lose weight, and fight to keep it off. Life is a journey. It is supposed to be enjoyed with ease and grace instead of fighting battles with your will power. When your will power is applied to weight loss, it doesn't work long term. Weight loss was a sixty-one-billion-dollar industry in 2010 according to Marketdata's 11th edition of the *U.S. Weight Loss & Diet Control Market* study. Over half the population is overweight and over 30 percent is morbidly obese. And more will join these sobering statistics in years to come.

I am always amazed by the countless ads running on TV promising the moon and the stars without your having to lift a finger. Even more amazing is the fact that people buy into that. What triggers these buying decisions? Is it desperation? Is it a lack of know-how or the lack of a role model? Is it instant gratification? Or a combination of these and/or other reasons? In the end, most people (the percentage ranges anywhere from 80 to over 90 percent depending on the source) who actually lose some weight gain it back again within three to five years, and many gain even more than they lost. A diet is just not sustainable. You have to come out of it at a certain point, and even if you want to, you can't deny or fight that urge to consume the very things that have been prohibited as if they were forbidden fruit. Diets are built on the assumption that your body is naturally weak and strong will power has to be exercised to force it to lose weight. But it is through innate wisdom that your body reaches its natural equilibrium.

I grew up in a time when and a place where being fat was not anything anyone could conjure up in their wildest of dreams, so the current mindset of going on diet after diet to lose weight strikes me as something very unnatural. I can relate to how and why it is happening because I was overweight myself because I was eating junky fast foods, burning the candle at both ends, gravitating to the couch too often, going after money for the wrong reasons, living for approval, and stressing myself to the core; I was living life from the outside for show. The extra weight was a by-product of that lifestyle, as were many other symptoms.

As you live a healthy lifestyle through a supporting mindset and good food choices, your body has the opportunity to build up more energy reserves from the ever-increasing good quality and quantity of your blood, while simultaneously producing enough organic energy to support you in all the activities you need to do on a daily basis. There is more energy for deep repair, restoration, and building a healthier body. The shift in consciousness shows you, either slowly or quickly, that everything that happens to you or with you is for you to experience. Every person you meet, whether you develop a relationship or simply cross paths, is there to either teach you a lesson or help you in some way on your soul's journey. Once you know and understand this, stress will not hold you down as it once did.

Your physical body is built for survival, intuitively keeping your soul safe and sound. Embracing this helps your mind perceive things in ways that support your body through its intricate, built-in mind-body hormonal messaging system. What separates us from other species is that we can live our way into youthfulness and vibrancy. It is understood that excessive weight is the combination of a sedentary lifestyle, poor eating habits, emotional bondage, and mind-induced stress. Living life whole and free allows excess weight to simply go away as a natural by-product of living a happy life.

- **Being at your ideal, natural, healthy weight:** Follow the daily bite-sized actions you will design and modify after reading *Young Mind Young Body*. They grow into you as part of life, become you and an extension of you, and grow with you until the day you are ready to drop your physical house and move on in your soul's journey. This ideal weight is where you feel most resilient, irresistible, young, energetic, happy, vibrant, enthusiastic, joyful, and vital. It is where your immunity is at peak level, effectively defending you from foreign invaders and viruses and offering you the chance to experience life in its entire splendor. You are fit and healthy-looking, with a natural body shape – strong, flexible, and slim, yet not frail. Again, this is the natural by-product of mindful and enjoyable living. There is hardly any need to count calories.

- **Being naturally high and able to lift yourself out of depression without antidepressants:** So many of us are silently suffering from depression, including those who seem to have it all. Robin McLaurin Williams (July 21, 1951 – August 11, 2014), the famous American actor and comedian who suffered from depression and committed suicide, comes to mind. When we live from the outside, life is very stressful. Worrying can easily become a habit when you're living with a "scarcity mindset" that makes you feel insecure, unsafe, and incomplete. Separating from the whole and stepping away from oneness make us feel lonely and in need of someone or something, and grabbing sugary things to eat and drink can make us feel marginally better while progressively driving us onto a roller coaster towards feeling depressed and unhappy. Depression is simply a by-product of stepping away from oneness.

By making a switch and journeying inward, you start to feel the oneness, the source, the abundance – the joy, happiness, peace, and forever. Superficial attachment to material things starts to lose its hold on you, as does being judgmental, angry, and unforgiving. You experience life as is. Life is not to be taken too seriously but experienced as different flavors. You choose the cast and characters that allow you to fully play this life out so you can live knowing you are perfect as is. When you get to the zone of highs, happiness flows out of you from the source and shows up on your face as light, as fire, as joy, and as your soul. Depression is a thing of the past.

The beauty of this is that it is all within you. All you need is the awareness, and then to simply learn to get in touch with your inner self that is a part of the universal whole, allowing the life spark to shine through in your unique way. You are so very high at times, often marveling at the magic of life and how fortunate it is to be alive. There are lows; there are highs. You build up your bodily strength to a point where there is enough energy to go around. Good circulation carries *qi* – life's vital energy – to your brain, keeping it at peak functioning and preventing the feeling of depression caused by fatigue due to insufficient air.

Cynthia, a level three reiki master and a friend and client of mine, recounted the bubbling sensations of joy and height she experienced in our tenth session together, five months into her six-month coaching program. She jokingly said that she had "reached Sue's level of high."

- **Feeling relaxed and calm:** One of the frequent comments I hear these days about me is that I am peaceful and calm. This was not how I showed up on the physical plane before I awakened and made meditation part of my routine. Life was chaotic, anything but peaceful. It was full of drama, stress, agitation, yelling, and screaming. I was desperate for something better, for someone to dig me out of my deep hole, for the greener grass in someone else's yard. It is this journey inward to home that has put me in this place of peace and calm and helped me relax into the very essence of being. This journey home started with physically healing from depression, desperation, being overweight, extreme fatigue, borderline diabetes, anger, resentment, and an aged face, body, mind, and heart – lost with no direction. It naturally extended to my mental, emotional, and spiritual healing and to actually living the life I wanted for myself. Over the years, at times I have still felt anger, but it's on the surface, not deep and shaking and debilitating as it was before, keeping me from doing anything other than "angry." Now I feel the same peace as in meditation, and easily juggle my busy life, my business, working with customers, building up my coaching practice, and being the mother of a preteen.

- **Being able to forgive:** Nelson Mandela said, "Resentment is like drinking poison and then hoping it will kill your enemies." Buddha, the ancient Indian philosopher and god figure, has often been quoted as saying "Holding on to anger is like grasping a hot coal with the intent of throwing it at someone else; you are the one who gets burned." The damaging effects of being angry and holding grudges and resentment have been proven. These emotions induce the harmful chemical hormones cortisol and adrenaline – the fight-or-flight stress hormones in the body – and create all sorts of physical disease. They cause indigestion, weight challenges, stress, and insomnia. They change your facial expressions and emanate negative energy and vibrations that bring about these negative traits. By living from the source, you foster a deeper understanding of who you are as a being and start seeing everything around you as parts of a whole. You begin to feel the oneness from source, from one another, slowly but surely coming to the knowing that everyone is part of you. By forgiving them, you forgive yourself. Forgiving is for me, for you, and for everyone else. It sets you free to pursue what is close to your heart by leaving space for new things to come in.

- **Letting go of the need to control, and allowing the infinite orchestrating power of the universe to take over and lift the heavy burden off your shoulders, leaving you lighthearted for moving forward:** I had been a worrier, and tried to compel things to happen in certain ways with certain results. It depressed and frustrated me when things did not go as planned, and I viewed myself as a failure. I know deeply what it is to feel debilitated by the worries and the expectations of others and of yourself, and to not be able to put any energy into the actual doing. By the end of the day, feelings of depression and hopelessness sink in, belittling the bravest person. There was a point in time when I was so overwhelmed that just the thought of all the things I needed to do sent me into a deep depression. Then it dawned on me that every moment of my life, regardless of what I had been doing, was part of my journey. There was no need to rush to be something different.

Once that realization registered, all the things I had heard, learned, and read, through being coached and coaching others, started to connect within, such as breaking projects down to easier-to-chew and digestible bite-sized chunks, and taking steady baby steps – one small step at a time, one thing at a time. When the feeling of overwhelm arises, I simply drop everything, take a deep breath, get centered, and start over fresh. The cultivated outlook that all is part of life and that everything happens in divine order has assisted me in moving into the here and now and the task at hand. It has been very helpful. I have a type-A personality, so I tend to pile up my plate with so much more than I can chew. I understand the value of focusing on the task at hand instead of being depleted from worrying and rushing. A type-A person is prone to running out of steam quickly if energy is not directed to where it counts the most.

By applying the comprehensive approach to building up youthful vitality, you are able to think with clarity and lay out action steps that come from the vision you hold for yourself for the life you dream of living. Then you act on it, step by step, with intensity in the here and now. Ingrain this approach in your daily habits and leave worrying out of the equation. The liberated feeling of lightness is very refreshing and the energy released is rejuvenating. It leaves you feeling young, vibrant, and full of vigor for a happy and prosperous life to be lived and embraced in the full awareness of now. All is possible. Once you allow things to happen the way they happen, you only need to give everything you are doing at hand your very best shot and not worry as to how it will turn out. In the end it is not in your hands. Many forces and variables play a part in it. Often, if you are open to the outcomes, they come out better than you could ever have imagined. It is as if the universe is at your side, delivering things just the way you are supposed to have them – at the right time, in the right amounts, in the right format, and with the right people. Allowing things to happen as they will leaves you to marvel that you could never have planned it out that way yourself and that the universe knows things you can't possibly know.

- **Feeling an increased sense of well-being and the joy of life:** When your energy is high and your health optimal, you are operating from the source, your life is balanced, and it is natural to have an increased sense of well-being. You feel so good at times you want to sing, dance, and shout to the world, "I LOVE YOU." You are connected with yourself in pure happiness and joy, and your bodily vitality fosters the feeling of being on top of the world, in your own skin, and being happy about it. This is the natural by-product of living life per design, using your regained, vibrant young mind and young body as your launching pad.

- **Living life with meaning and purpose:** You are here to fulfill your desires and wishes, to live through certain experiences, to realize the perfect being you are, to realize you have had it all as a spiritual being but have to experience the imperfection to see the perfection. You came to this world with sets of talents to accommodate those desires, sustaining yourself while serving the world at large so that you live with zest, fire, and drive. Purpose is the original source of life, and is replenished time after time by your "charge center" when it is aligned perfectly in sync with the cosmic design. You know this when your professional life and your personal life merge as one with no distinction between fun and work. You don't even think about whether you are working or having fun; you simply leave it to others to decide. But the fire is there, easy to see and identify in the way you do things, the manner in which you speak, and the way your eyes sparkle with everyone you meet and everything you touch and everything you do. You glow like light, smiling to yourself often, causing others to ask, "What is all that smiling about?" You reply, "Don't know. Don't care. I'm simply happy."

Of course, this way of living is adding more years to your life and more life to your years! You want to eat better for your body, sleep better to build more quality blood and good *qi,* and move your body more to increase your body mass, muscle tone, bone density, and heart capacity. This, in turn, makes you happier, healthier, and wanting everyone else to have the young mind and young body that you have, feel the same way you feel about life, and spread the joy of simply being alive. Others catch that uplifting energy and vibration that you naturally emanate. By being you, you are raising mother earth's happy vibration! That energy comes back to you and raises you even higher! What a self-fulfilling prophecy! How beautiful can it be!

- **Experiencing growth and expansion in all areas of life:** How else would it be except prospering in all areas of life when you live this way? We traditionally view success as the accumulation of material wealth – money and things that represent status, not giving much value to living life happily. Consequently so many of us approach life with a priority of having a good-paying job that shows status and material success. Then comes a time when we hate what we do but feel trapped with a family to support, a status quo to maintain, bigger and bigger mortgages to pay, cars to maintain, a standard of living to keep up with… on and on. Even though we grow to hate our profession or business, we force ourselves to stay at it day in and day out, year in and year out, until we get burned out and physically break down with fatigue, weight gain, and diabetes. We experience built-up resentment and feel sorry and depressed. We wonder what life is all about with no pleasure but only bills to pay and responsibilities to keep up.

The way to approach a successful life is to be a successful *person* first. Live life happy and fulfilled from deep within, doing the things your heart calls you to do that best showcase what makes you shine, your talents, and your passion – the whole package. Money, fame, better relationships, better sleep, better health, and feeling better come as by-products. That's why some people seem to have everything right while others seem to have everything working against them. Success is in that flow, whether it's to your benefit or working against you, and you are the creator of it all. Once you start building up your health and youth with a vibrant young mind and young body, you set the stage for success to fall into place.

After many years of unmindful living it can take many years of mindful living to undo the negative results. Stay with it, don't rush it, and let it run its course. In the meantime, you are enjoying the process. You are learning and understanding the full scope of how life works, evolves, and straightens itself out. Now that the foundation is solidly built, you are on a rising trend with the intention to be in sync and in alignment with the inner truth of that which you are. Stay with that truth, firmly grounded in it, not to be derailed by any outside force.

- **Enjoying a boosted immunity, therefore being sick less and bouncing back quickly whenever sick:** This is one of the most important benefits of putting the proper lifestyle habits into place and practicing them consistently. It takes six months to a year depending on where you were at the time you started. Now that you are doing the right things, your body automatically starts building itself up. When extra blood is made available, your body knows what repairs need to be done first on top of keeping its daily functions going with everything you have on your plate. It's wise to do everything in your power to help your body with these deep repairs by eating right, getting enough quality sleep in the right time period, and moving often to keep your muscles and bones strong to efficiently metabolize food. Stay happy and relaxed and avoid things that unnecessarily deplete your precious energy. Soon your consumption of energy is less than the amount of energy you generate on a daily basis so that you start to build up energy reserves. You no longer burn your energy reserves putting your body in the stage of inflamed yin. Youthful vigor returns to you in full swing, making you want to dance, sing, and skip a few steps when walking. You are sick less often, and should you get sick, it is of a much shorter duration and lesser severity. Proper self-care and self-love are critical in keeping you in this phase of health building.

- **Being able to enjoy longevity and good quality of life:** It is one thing to live a long life. It is quite another to live long in vibrant health and be happy. It is widely known that people who live mindfully and make supporting mindset, lifestyle, and food choices have much better odds of enjoying long, quality lives. I was told by a bookstore owner in Chicago's Chinatown that the senior community home there had many centenarians. One resident complained to her that he was over eighty, yet he had not earned the privilege of having a birthday party hosted in his honor because he was too young. Only the centenarians had earned that.

Dan Buettner, a cyclist, educator, speaker, and embodiment of youth, well preserved at age fifty-five, authored a book, *The Blue Zones: Lessons for Living Longer from the People Who've Lived the Longest*. The book details the five areas in the world where the population enjoys an average lifespan of about ten years longer than Americans and those in Western European countries. It is clear to me that these people share something in common: a healthy lifestyle. They eat what is being produced locally, stay active, live in harmony with their natural environment, and rest well. They also seem to enjoy the community they live in and go with life's flow with leisure, ease, and happiness. You don't need to move there to benefit from their way of life. You are bringing these qualities into your own life.

There are more and more people enjoying the fruits of a long life being lived to the fullest. Just be mindful and fully aware of the choices you make in the here and now. It can be something small and insignificant, such as adding more greens to your diet, taking a walk, and going to bed early and getting up early, or something that requires you to apply yourself, like learning not to worry; deciding to be happy; being gentle, kind, and loving to yourself; and saying things that are self-supportive and not self-diminishing. It does take some awareness and conscious choice-making in the beginning. But once you have done it for a while, your brain is rewired and new grooves and new patterns form. Then your new habits become automatic. Living your best life possible, with ease and grace, is not a trying effort any longer. First making conscious choices, and then embodying them in daily life, is the key to maintaining your new way of life.

- **Enjoying more clarity in thinking, therefore making better decisions:** I remember the days when I was overweight, bitter, depressed, and feeling sick – my brain couldn't function well either. Something blocked me from thinking clearly. I could not even finish reading a sentence without forgetting the beginning of it, nor could I comprehend. Many of the poor choices made during those years were partially due to unclear thinking. That state of sluggish mind-functioning was a consequence of the total unhealthy package that accompanied the life I was leading back then. I was ungrounded and derailed from the truth of who I was, running around, spinning like a hamster on a wheel. I have been gaining clearer thinking ever since I started cleaning up my food intake, making more supporting lifestyle choices, getting in touch with my true reality, building up my bodily reserves, and making choices aligned with my deepest wishes and desires that are guided by my gut intuition. I often marvel at the way I feel in my head now: clean, vibrant, and clear, with no blockages. I had never really experienced that in my life before. Now that you are on your healing journey, sharper brain capacity and better decision-making are side effects of conscious living.

- **Developing a sense of unity, oneness, and belongingness:** By living in alignment with nature and going within, you slowly but surely start sensing the oneness, the unity, and being part of a whole. Now that you are feeling that, it is so much easier to be kinder, gentler, and nicer to yourself and your fellow beings, even if some of them are hard to comprehend. You look at everyone with love, compassion, and understanding, knowing they are here just as you to experience life for a higher purpose.

- **Feeling bolder, more authentic, and more aligned with your core essence:** You start to act from your center in your own unique way, in your voice, in your facial expression, and in your body language, with your unique talent that no one else is ever made to match. Once you understand your authenticity, you start to possess what is called *personal power* – that of your true self, as opposed to *agency power,* which is power from something else to make you look superficially bigger. You understand that diminishing your divine gifts is doing an injustice to mankind. By hiding, downsizing your dreams, thinking that you are not enough, and skipping on the surface of life, you were wasting away. Now you can start to own your gift, step up to the plate, stand in your own light, and shine your shine for the world around you to benefit one way or another. Or you might simply show the world that spark of universal light shining through you, igniting other lights to shine where your light permeates.

- **Being more loving, lovable, forgiving, and grateful, and growing a sense of abundance:** These are the qualities you see in people you admire – the people who seem to have everything together. People love to be around them. They exuberate love, gentleness, understanding, forgiving, grace, and a sense of having it all. Some just grew up in an environment like that, with parents or grandparents having these qualities. For most of us they are learned qualities, with awareness as a start. Now that you are on this journey of self-discovery with an open heart and an open mind, ready to take in what is, you gradually become more of your essence. Love shines through, showing up in your physical world. You take life as a gift, living it with appreciation and grace. On your way there, abundance finds you. It knocks on your door. There is only love and its embodiment in abundance.

- **Being more at ease and able to follow the flow of life:** Surely life doesn't need to be a struggle, which doesn't mean you won't struggle at all anymore; it only means you focus your efforts on where you want your life to head instead of being disabled by worries. You learn to show up, co-create with the creator, and go with the flow of life – downstream sailing instead of upstream fighting. All too often we call life a fight or a battleground. It does not need to be a fight. It can be a game played with fun and joy. It can be a symphony, with lows and highs, and you can simply dance through it all. It is your take on life that matters in the end. You could be doing the same things as seen from the outside, but your true reality lies in the way you perceive life. This reality has a big impact on your health and well-being, and you either build yourself up or deplete yourself depending on the reality you choose for yourself.

- **Being more adept at dealing with life's ups and downs:** Now that you have come to the realization that life is all about experiencing experiences, you view the ups and downs differently. They are meant to initiate meaningful insights and wake up the knowing you have within you. Truly live your experiences instead of simply knowing. Your regained youth and vitality, stemming from the building up of energy reserves by following a supporting lifestyle routine, also make you more adept at taking life as it comes.

I am sure you know what it feels like when you are healthy and energetic. The hurdles in life don't seem as daunting as they did when you were feeling tired, stressed out, worn out, and depressed, with many bodily burdens to boot. You really have to experience this state of being to appreciate its implications in your happiness. Happiness is a feeling; it's very elusive, but it can be obtained through tangible living and made available to you through your choices.

Chapter Two

Erase the Detrimental Effects of Life's Stress

Millions of years of evolution and adaptation have developed the way our human bodies respond to stress, with sympathetic stress response and parasympathetic relaxation response. In the sympathetic stress response, or the fight-or-flight response, your brain sets off an alarm system in your body when you face a threat, perceived or real. Through an intricate combination of nerve and hormonal signals, this mechanism signals your adrenal glands to release a flood of hormones such as adrenaline and cortisol. These hormones increase your heart or pulse rate and raise your blood pressure to boost energy supplies to prepare you to fight or run. Meanwhile, digestion and assimilation of food stop working because life is in danger. When our hunter-gatherer ancestor saw a tiger approaching, blood would be shunted from their gut to their brain to think fast for surviving, and to their legs and arms to pump them up either to fight battles or run away from the threatening danger. Once the danger was over, the body returned to normal.

Nowadays most of us worry too much about money, health, future security, body image, and relationships. Some worries are real, but most are perceived only in the mind. Even though these are mind-induced stresses, different from the physical threats of fight or flight, our bodies respond to them the same way. What makes them more detrimental is that we can't give it a good fight, release the stresses, and get it over with. The stress response is constantly on, which triggers more adrenaline, cortisol, and insulin secretion. This, in turn, drives weight gain, the onset of type II diabetes, and much other stress-related "dis-ease," aging and heart attacks included. It was reported in a Gallup survey that Monday mornings are when the highest rates of hospital emergencies from stress-induced heart attacks occur. It is also stated in the "Heart Attack Statistics" at AllHeartAttack.com that studies show the most common time for a heart attack is Monday morning. Why is that? Maybe because so many of us are so stressed out that after a weekend away from work just the idea of going back to the places we hate so much causes our hearts to give out.

My sister is very active, fit, and trim. She eats wholesome, mostly plant-based foods. Financially she is not wealthy by the conventional definition, but she has everything she needs to live comfortably. Yet like so many people around her, she worried so much about being taken care of in her old age that she developed short-term memory issues. With so much stress coming from the fear and insecurity, the brain cells associated with short-term memory were damaged, causing her to forget tasks at hand. This almost caused their house to catch fire.

A friend told me that she couldn't stop worrying, especially late at night, and had a hard time falling asleep. Even if she had nothing to worry about, she would come up with something to worry about – the what-ifs – "What will I do if such-and-such happens?"

I, too, suffered tremendously from the what-ifs, partly resulting from endless worries about money and not having enough business. What would happen if my competitors took all my business away? What if I were unable to provide a secure future for myself and my family? What if I were unable to send my daughter to college? Sometimes I didn't even know what all the worries and stress were about; it was just sort of a general way of living, being, thinking, and behaving. Then, of course, my body bore the burdens of that kind of thinking. I struggled through each day without being able to enjoy life or savor, taste, and experience from deep within.

Everyday stress has driven many people into early graves. It is associated with all the modern-day epidemics out there: heart disease, cancer, diabetes, obesity, memory loss, fatigue, and so on. If you can learn to erase the stress in your life and turn on the parasympathetic relaxation response more often, you will have very good odds of being much younger, both in body and mind. You will enjoy the vibrancy that comes with youth because your body will be relaxed and your digestion will be working well to assimilate foods. Life will be peaceful and full of sunshine and magic. Here are the steps for erasing stress:

1. Make Time Your Ally

By time, I mean clock time, indicated by man-made machines, to reference things. Everyone has the same time in any given day: twenty-four hours a day. So instead of competing with time, make time your ally and be a leisurely person. It is possible even if you are very busy. All it requires is a shift in perception. Regardless of how you look at time or how you rush, there is not much you can do about gaining more time for yourself. All you are doing is gaining yourself more aging from the pressure you put on yourself by pushing yourself too hard. "Haste makes waste" still applies. There is a sign at a cemetery site that says, "Don't rush. We can wait." Does that make sense to you? You don't need to rush through life and drive yourself to an early death. You can just take it easy and live life. Do things along the lines of the following to make time your ally and escape its hold on you:

- Leave yourself enough time so you don't feel the pressure to rush.
- Invite a friend for tea to catch up on things.
- Call a friend whom you have lost touch with for a while, for no apparent reason.
- Cook something you crave.
- Garden.
- Stop and smell the roses.
- Enjoy your lunch, sitting down, with no rush.

- Read a book that speaks to you.
- Walk and commune with nature.
- Stroke your cat or walk your dog.
- Play with your kids.
- Have at least one day to yourself, with no scheduling.
- Golf or fish, if they appeal to you.
- Hike.
- Drive at a normal speed. If someone is in a hurry, let him or her pass instead of getting angry about it. All too often you find them right in front of you, waiting at the traffic light, leaving you wondering what all that rushing was about.
- Make a not-to-do list instead of a to-do list. Take out the junky, rushed activities that are clogging your daily life, like some of the parties that go nowhere, or your kids' extra after-school activities.
- The dishes can wait till tomorrow; I bet they won't be running out on you if you don't wash them today.

You will be able to find time to pull out of the fast lane if you realize how detrimental the fast lane is. It is almost as if on one end you are trying to gain some momentum, only to lose it at the other end by being sick or dying early. Sometimes you might even start to wonder what the point is. There really is no point. Everything can wait, if you allow it. It comes down to how much you value yourself and your health. It is when you slow down that you might start to gain momentum by only focusing on the things that matter to you, from deep within.

2. Live in the Here and Now

"All things exist in the Now, including the past, present, and future; this is the true meaning of the Eternal Moment," says Bruce Adams, author of *Prophet or Madman* (p. 120).

Everything happens in the here and now, either past or future; the past is the past here and now while the future is a future here and now – nonetheless a here and now. We tend to dwell on the past, giving it romance, color, and wishful thinking. Then we worry a lot about the future – about how things are going to turn out, what our lives will be like, how we are going to be provided for in our old age, where the country is going to go, how the world is going to be fed – on and on. In the meantime, we miss out on living in the here and now, which is the only tangible we've got. When you regret or resent or get lost in wishful thinking, you are living in the past; things happened that you can do nothing about. When you worry, you are traveling into the future, since the future is not here and will never be here. The worries are pretty much mind-induced, resulting from the separation from oneness – walking away from the source and from one another.

Present-moment awareness is very powerful in shaping your future. By not living in it, you rob yourself of the precious gift of experiencing life to the fullest, with all that entails. Present-moment awareness connects you with your essence, enabling you to understand yourself as the being you are. Alice Morse Earle once wrote, "Yesterday is history. Tomorrow is a mystery. Today is a gift. That's why it's called the present." To truly live life the way your heart desires, you only need to focus on present-moment awareness and the present task at hand. When you live in the now, you catch anything that is surfacing from mind-induced toxic emotions. You can then assimilate it immediately, leaving no residue.

One time I was with my friend Harry, chatting in a car parked in a peaceful area where leaves gently whispered the beauty of life, telling the story of peace and eternity on a colorful and vibrant autumn day. I talked with him about the moment, which brought him back from worrying about the future of his business to that special moment, appreciating the beauty, bounty, and harmony of life surrounding us all. Not too long ago, he told me of that particular day, with the rustling of leaves singing the songs of a beautiful and harmonious fall day, and how he kept thinking of that moment when he felt he was being pulled off center in all different directions, and how remembering that moment brought him back to the here and now.

Tantra, an ancient East Indian religion and life philosophy, says intensity is the only thing needed to know the truth. That intensity can be obtained by dropping the past and letting go of the future. Thus your whole life energy is directed to the small here and now. In that focusing, you are a fire, ready to set the world on fire. When you carry the past, much of your life force is diverted to the past – a past that is not. When you worry about the future, much of your energy is diverted to the future – not yet here, waiting to be shaped by your here-and-now actions made aware.

Lao Tzu, in the classic Chinese text *Tao Te Ching,* says, "One who lives in accordance with nature does not go against the way of things. He moves in harmony with the present moment, always knowing the truth of just what to do."

When you eat, eat. Take time savoring your three meals. When you meditate, meditate. When you do yoga, focus on your stretches. When you practice qigong, allow your moves to follow your intention and coordinate your breathing. When you drive, pay full attention to the driving. When you work, give the tasks at hand your very best. When you walk, take it all in. When you garden, garden with your whole person. When you read, read with the totality of which you are. When you play with your kids, be there with them 100 percent. When spending time with a loved one, immerse in it. When listening to a friend who desperately needs your attentive ear, give your friend both your ears. When you brainstorm about the business of your heart's desire, be in that moment with an open heart and mind and the wholesome approach that carries your soul. By being in the here and now, you are shaping your future with a constant awareness, becoming the co-creator of your destiny instead of a victim of circumstance.

Only visit and reflect on the past to the extent of lessons to be learned, and only evaluate the future when making plans – maybe a total of 10 to 20 percent of your clock time. The rest of the time stay grounded in the here and now.

The past is long gone, and the future is not yet here, waiting for you to shape it with your present-moment presence, intention, attention, and actions. That is the only way to live life with no regrets, no wishful thinking, no hiding, no what-ifs; but with aliveness, happiness, contentment, and fulfillment. When things get seemingly tough and painful, it's not always easy to stay in the present moment. It does take constant awareness and understanding to live in the moment of now instead of regretting the past, dreaming, and flying into the future. Keep in mind that focusing on the present moment is the only way to face your life head-on, dissolve undissolved emotions, and fully experience and assimilate life's experiences. By avoiding living in the current moment, you are robbing your soul's intention of fully experiencing life, whatever it might be. So make a pact with it; let it be okay if it is too painful. Observe the urge to hide behind busyness by staying superficially busy, and to hide behind numbness by watching TV and skipping on the surface of life without really living it fully. Do not exercise judgment while observing.

When you catch yourself drifting away from the present moment, simply get back into it again – it is that moment, when you are aware that you are not in the here and now in your body, that you are present with yourself. If the emotion gets too painful, simply allow yourself to feel the emotion while you silently observe. By honoring that emotion with space and attention, you are dissolving it into thin air and healing yourself from deep within. By witnessing yourself in the act of experiencing the emotions, you are disassociating yourself from the emotions you are experiencing. You will come to know that you are not your emotions, and they cannot run your life. You are way above and beyond your emotions. You are so much more.

Be ready to embrace life's presents, gifts, messages, surprises, and guidance. Experience dreams being fulfilled, desires being manifested in the physical realm, wisdom being gained, and aha! moments being tucked away like treasures found while walking on the beach. Remain open and relaxed. Allow life in! It is your life; live it as you please by being fully immersed in the here and now.

3. Embrace You and Your Life As Is

The grass is always greener in others' yards. It is almost second nature to compare yourself with others – the way you look, the house you live in, your job, the college your kids go to, the car you drive, etc. You are so busy comparing that you overlook the fact that everything is the way it is supposed to be. In the end, nothing matters except the soul's journey, along with the assimilation of your experiences – emotionally, spiritually, mentally, and physically. How often do you wish you were in someone else's life, seeing the glamour, success, and all that comes with it? The thing you are not seeing is the story behind the scene. I recently saw a telling picture of a ballerina's feet. The right foot was for the stage and was in a beautiful ballet shoe while the left foot was an off-stage view, with bruises all over it. It just goes to show that you often see only half of the story.

One time I heard a business owner complaining about how useless it was to have been in business for over ten years without any major growth. A friend of his had been in business for a short three years and had constant online orders from numerous representatives, and his business was hustling and buzzing with activity. I am not against a business being big or having sales; on the contrary, I always look for ways to increase my exposure. The point is that my friend was so bitter and beaten that he considered himself useless. He was discrediting the fact of being in business for so many years and showing a profit and supporting his family and his own sustaining power.

True, it would be nice to be able to magically expand your business and quadruple your income. You can be on top of the world right this very moment if you so choose. All you need to do is simply accept you and your life for what they are and appreciate the fact that you are what you are and your life is what it is. Remember that it can always be better, and it can always be worse. There is no use in comparing. There are always going to be people who are doing so much better, who look so much better, if you really want to make yourself feel miserable. On the other hand, there are always going to be people who do not look nearly as good as you look, and who are far less fortunate than you are.

It is when you accept who you are and the way your life is that you give yourself permission to be happy with life. You can move forward in life burden-free, with a lighter body and heart, spreading your waves of energy and light while you merrily hop along. It is as if by magic you start to attract more of the quality and the things you dream of having in your life while you enjoy your life, carefree. This is called LIKES ATTRACT LIKES, the cosmic law of attraction at work. It is essential to start to embrace you and your life the way they are.

It pays to have a good understanding of the nature of things, what Buddha practiced as *suchness.* It is winter; it is cold; it is what is. You have debt that is from years of impulsive behaviors; what is done is done; there is nothing you can do about it except address it in the here and now. You cannot go back and change what you did over the decades; it is what is. If the sun is blazing hot on a hot afternoon, complaining is not going to change it; such is the nature of things. When you accept, you are on top of the world. If you accept because you have to, you will be continually in pain and suffering. When you accept without any complaint – not because you have no other choice but only because you understand, suchness happens. You have the choice to accept like a beggar, or like a queen or a king. The difference is huge between a life of misery, failure, and hardship and one of happiness, success, and ease. The choice always remains yours.

Haven't you seen enough of desperate people struggling their way out of their ruts but ending up sinking deeper, being more miserable and bitter? They carry around with them a huge pull of negative energy that you can smell from miles away. What they don't get is that all they need to do is just be happy for what they are. Once someone asked a wiser person, "How can I be happy if I am homeless?" The wiser person replied, "You should be happy that you do not have a mortgage to pay, as do so many people, struggling day in and day out to pay their mortgage."

Body image is an issue for many people, like "I wish my legs were longer," "my hair was fuller," "my face more beautiful," "my nose higher," etc. It all begins to get better with self-acceptance. True, you can't change your physical attributes, but you can for sure change the way you feel about them. By simply accepting yourself for whatsoever you are, you announce to the world that you are enough and that you love yourself for what you are, however you are. With that acceptance comes the glow from within. Suddenly you become radiant. Watch how the world responds to that energy. The world will fall in love with you simply because you emit a love vibration for that which you are. That truth resonates with the truth that lies in every one of us.

So how do you go about doing it on a daily basis? For starters, stare at yourself in the mirror every day telling yourself the reflection in the mirror is the house with which you came equipped into this world. You chose to have that face, that body, and certain life experiences. So be okay with it. It is the way you are supposed to look. Appreciate that face, have compassion and love for it. Keep in mind that this appreciation and acceptance shows up on your face as radiance, confidence, and contentment. These show up as a glow on your face to compensate for much of the plainness you might think you have.

Second, be okay with where you are in your life. It is good wherever you are. It is the place you are supposed to be. So make peace with it, even though your life might not be what you envisioned it being. This is the first step in having the life of your dreams. There is a Chinese saying that goes, "Thousands of miles start with the first step." Totally being okay with the way your life is right at this moment is the very first step towards attracting the life you have been dreaming of. Pat yourself on the shoulder for your braveness to have come this far, to be where you are, and to be experiencing all the flavors of life and enjoying life's abundance.

Third, catch yourself whenever you find yourself unconsciously comparing yourself to others, whether it is your body, your house, your job, or your business. Tell yourself that things are the way they are supposed to be, even though it is quite beneficial to learn from others, as a business equipped with a long-term vision aligned with the founder's deepest purpose, passion, and dream.

4. Prioritize Your Life

I once had a to-do list because many of the gurus out there said it was the only way to be sure things get done. But all too often I found myself depressed, looking at the things that needed to be done, to a point that it was almost impossible to move ahead in life. It might work for some people, and it worked for me sometimes, but I have since realized that the best way to really make headways in life is to focus on doing that one thing that is most important to me – that something that makes my heart sing, my blood run faster, my creative juices flow; that something that puts a glow on my face, deeply knowing that I am doing something that feeds my heart and soul, like the book I am writing at this very moment, sitting at my desk with nothing else planned except writing for about one hour. That leaves me enough time to get my online posting done and breakfast ready for the family, and be ready, mentally and physically, for the day. The rest can all wait. I have found it unnecessary to do certain things anymore, and I am not heartbroken for leaving them undone.

I know from firsthand experience how easy it is to feel overwhelmed, stuck on the tracks, stressed out, feeling old and beaten inside out and outside in. Everyone, including you and me, has the same time, 24/7 per clock time. The difference between those with fulfilling lives and those who are spinning wheels and beating themselves senseless is that the former are living with a priority originating from their deepest desire.

Think about what is really important to you. What makes your heart sing? What makes you happy or excited? How would you like your life to be in five years, ten years, twenty years, or even on the day you decide to leave your physical house? Meditate on these questions and observe your responses. Once you know what it is that you really want to get done in this lifetime, break things down into bite-sized pieces. Then take baby steps and be sure to do a little every day, just like the writing I am doing now. With the help of Christine Kloser's Get Your Book Done program, I broke the impossibly overwhelming task of writing a book into many easy-to-assimilate bite-sized pieces and felt deeply satisfied. I made headway towards something so special and meaningful. If I drifted away a bit, I simply got right back at it where I left off.

Once you focus on what is important to you, act on concentrating the bulk of your presence, intention, attention, thoughts, and actions on it. You will find yourself having ample time for it by letting go of the things that are not so essential yet drain your emotion and energy. It is not serving you well to just keep being a busy bee, blindly meeting deadlines, beating yourself senseless, and doing everything that comes your way.

Give yourself some quiet time. Sit with things. Ponder things through. Talk things over with your family, friends, those in your circle of influence, and, if necessary, a coach. Come up with a clear picture or idea of your priorities in life. Then brainstorm the actions or action steps needed to start the project of your life. Get rid of all the clutter in your life, including emotional blocks, made-up stories, and attachments to certain results or expectations. Keep at it, a little at a time. Whenever the feeling of stress and overwhelm hits you, simply get back to your center and realign. You can move mountains with this clarity and focus on priority.

5. Live with Gratitude

When you live life with gratitude, your ego leaves a way for your true self to shine through, enabling you to live with grace. You genuinely feel grateful for everything and everyone. That energy, in turn, attracts more of the quality you desire in your life. We all know of people who take everything for granted, demanding things to be their way as if the world owes them. This attitude has contributed to much of the so-called social injustice in the world. I understand circumstances play roles in people's lives, and we all need help from one another at one time or another. Some need more than others. The elderly, children, and sick people need the most care from society as a whole. We are all obligated to help those who are in need since we are all part of the whole.

Gratitude is a way of being. It shifts your perspective. It allows you to remain humble and to respond to life in a more graceful way. It offers you the space of giving yourself permission to be happy with what is and pleasantly surprised at life's happenings and the people who cross your path, offering you experiences and opportunities you never knew existed. Learn to be grateful for everything that happens in your life and for every person you encounter, whether they are the very person you need at that moment in your life or someone there to simply deliver a message, guide your way, or show you a part of you and make you understand yourself better.

Here are a few practical tips you can apply to foster a grateful way of living life:

- Every morning, right after you awake, sit up right where you sleep with eyes closed. Immerse yourself in the blessings of your life and inventory everything that counts. Be grateful that you woke up to another day with all it entails and the endless possibilities. Be grateful you are fortunate enough to be alive, even though you might not think your life is as you envisioned. Remember that you are fortunate enough to be able to experience life whatever way it is. Some people are forced to leave this life without it being their own conscious choice. Being alive is a beautiful thing. Be thankful for the fact that your body has evolved and adapted to evolution, bringing you to where you are today, being able to breathe in life's vital energy. Be grateful for the bed that has given you a night's restful, restorative sleep, and the roof over your head that protects you from bitter cold and harmful elements. Be grateful for the free air that is the cosmic life force. Be grateful for the people in your life, especially for those always on your side regardless of how moody, irritable, demanding, or careless you are – those who care about you whether you are dressed up or dressed down, whether you make money or not, whether you are successful in the traditional sense or down on your knees seeking life's answers and praying for miracles. The list goes on.

Gratitude comes from within. It shines past your ego's agenda of victim mentality, greediness, and expecting too much from others and the world around you. When you learn to be grateful, a subtle mindset shift occurs, rewiring your brain by forming new grooves. It becomes a natural habit to be thankful for every person crossing your path, even those you find irritating. Your heart bursts with gratitude for even the smallest of things in life. A happiness glow shines through you, brightening up your life, drawing more people to you, and inspiring those who want to build you up. You smile ear to ear, all day long, without even knowing you are smiling. It becomes a feature of you, radiating from within.

- During the day, be thankful for every person you meet, even for those who seem troublesome to you. Trust that anything that happens to you is for you and your further evolution. Learn to look at everything from this perspective. Sooner or later, probably sooner than you think possible, you view things from this inner place, taking nothing for granted. This gradually moves you out of being the victim, blaming all the so-called misfortunes on everyone but yourself. You begin to take charge of your life and become the co-creator of your destiny.

- Before going to bed, find a quiet place, reflecting again on your day, saying a silent thank you to the force behind all that is and the coincidences that happened during the day. Marvel at the way the universe operates: as if by some magic you have been carried along on the evolutional tide as part of the cosmic dance.

In the beginning, you might find it hard to find anything for which to be grateful, considering the social conditioning imposed upon you. Reflect on all the things you depend on; without them, you wouldn't be able to survive and smell the richness of life. For example, the people who deliver your mail, the farmers who grow your food, the distributors and transportation companies who make food available at your local stores, the convenience of life being delivered to you, day in and day out, without your ever thinking about it. Start marveling at everything in your life and your relationship of sustaining and thriving with everything, such as the coach who transformed your life, the article that shed light on the importance of eating habits and lifestyle choices, the taxi driver who just mumbled something to you on your way to the airport, turning on one of your switches instantly. Before long you will have a long list of all the things you would normally be taking for granted, thinking, "Yep, I have paid for it, and I deserve it." Granted, these are exchanges of energy in the form of goods and money, but they do serve you in the end, especially when you get life-sustaining value from them.

Think of this scenario: You get stuck in the desert with money, but nothing life-sustaining available. Now imagine a vendor in that life-threatening place selling water and food. I bet you would be so very grateful for his presence that you would give everything you had in exchange for his service.

If you think life is unfair to you, and you have nothing to be thankful for, thank the free air you are breathing for keeping you alive and the free sunshine for warming your skin, whether you think yourself deserving or not. There is always something, someone, to be thankful for in your life: a book, a teacher, a dream, your husband, your wife, your kids, your cat that is purring in your arms or sleeping on your desk while you type on your computer, the local farmer who sells organic produce at the farmer's market. Even if you are homeless, God forbid, then you do not have the responsibility of a mortgage and all the other costs associated with housing. You are temporarily bill-free. Learn to make a habit of reflecting on all the things that make your life more enjoyable and your experience more unique.

A long-term gratitude practice, like any other routine building, remaps the brain to respond with gratefulness as a built-in response, subtly shifting the mind to be less needy, more secure, and more abundant, therefore reducing the unnecessary stress associated with battling and struggling.

6. Adopt the "Abundance Principle"

When I walk around my neighborhood, I find apple trees and walnut trees bearing tremendous amounts of fruits, covering the ground around them. It seems no one picks them or enjoys them, besides the animals that munch on some of them. I see homeowners shoveling perfectly good walnuts into trash cans. I often wonder about the abundance of this fertile land and the huge waste. A classmate of mine from my college days in China – a professor now, visited me a few summers back. I took her to our 5.6-acre property, thinking she was going to comment on the messiness, plainness, and insignificance of the place. I was taken by surprise when she said we were so rich and lucky to have such a place. The next thing out of her mouth was even more surprising: what a waste that we were just letting it sit idle without planting something useful like vegetables, fruit trees, or even straight trees that could be used for building houses.

It puzzles me why most people buy commercial apples, which lab tests have shown bear the most chemical residues, instead of eating organic apples produced in their own yards or found along the road. Is it concern for trespassing for those who do not own the trees or is it that it has never occurred to most of us to eat something that is freely given by our mother earth? Or is it because the apples are too buggy? America is still the country with the most resources and the wealthiest by any standard. Why are most people working so hard, worrying so much, and putting so much stress and pressure on themselves? It never seems to be enough. The bigger houses, newer and better cars, and endless possessions seem to be dragging most of us down. What is it that most of us are searching for? Will outside abundance bring us happiness and satisfaction inside? Once we are there, will we feel the happiness and satisfaction we set out to have?

I was in this trap for many years, driving myself crazy, collecting houses, working on a business my heart was not in, day in and day out for over a decade, sick and lost in the process. In my quest for a life with more meaning and purpose, I found the magic of living life with gratitude. I came to the realization that abundance cannot be completely found from the outside environment. We have been put on this miraculous earth with an abundance of sunshine, rain, and air, which in turn produces an abundance of fruits, vegetables, grains, and wild game. This abundance can nourish us as the beings we are and support us in living the lives we are born to live.

It is a choice to either harvest the abundance all around you or feel deprived or victimized. It is the difference between a life filled with joy, happiness, and a sense of well-being, and a life of bitterness and struggle. For most of us living in this day and age, it takes a shift in consciousness and perception. Do you ever imagine that happiness could be this close, within reach, a matter of a shift? The truth is, it is that simple.

Most of us are born into this life with everything we will ever need to be happy and content. Our basic needs have been taken care of, first by our caretakers, then by ourselves through energy exchange. We attract things and people that emanate energy that matches the energy vibrations of our core being. All we need to do is trust the natural order of things; go through life with gratitude, detachment from rewards, mindfulness, and effortless grace; and do what is asked of us or that which requires our special imprint. Abundance follows as the natural flow of things. Stressful living, such as what most of us experience now, is not necessary at all. It is a by-product of our creation, originating from the mindset of separation and lack.

Enjoy the abundance that is all around you: the lushness of greens, the warmth and brightness of sunshine, the bounty of nature, love, gracefulness, your health, your good fortune, and the pure joy of being. Gratitude and abundance go hand in hand. For today, meditate on the phrase "Gratitude is for me. Gratitude draws abundance in my life."

7. Choose Supporting Perspectives

One time my peer coach asked me what my view of "perspective" was. I realized my view of perspective by itself was a perspective. Some people say perspective is everything. Some say it is how you look at things. When my daughter was ten, she said to me, "It is all about opinions." What is your perspective on perspective?

I found these descriptions of perspective on the internet:

1. The art of drawing solid objects on a two-dimensional surface so as to give the right impression of their height, width, depth, and position in relation to each other when viewed from a particular point; a perspective drawing

2. A particular attitude towards or way of regarding something; a point of view. Synonyms: outlook, view, viewpoint, point of view, standpoint, position, stand, stance, angle, attitude, frame of mind, frame of reference, approach, way of looking, interpretation, etc.

It looks like perspective is highly subjective, depending on a person's circumstances. Different people can have different perspectives on the same thing. For example, today is beautiful with nice sunshine, a little above 70°F. One person says, "How beautiful it is today; not too hot, not too cold." While another complains, "I love it really hot." And yet another, "It is kind of windy, though." Don't we all see lots of that going on in our lives? Interesting, right? You can see that there are as many perspectives as there are people. Even you view the same things differently at different times of the day or during different phases of your life.

That is the beauty of life. It is often not black or white, right or wrong, but just a point of view. So you don't need to take anything too seriously. Some say we all come equipped with a sixth sense – the sense of humor. Somehow your soul decided to come here to experience the life it chose to experience, but once it got into human form it all but forgot about the original plan. All the people appearing in your life are just like a cast of characters, helping you fulfill your soul's destiny. So the next time you feel you are being fooled or being cheated out of something, laugh it off, reminding yourself it is no big deal. Instead, thank the person who has to perform this nasty task for your soul's evolutional benefit.

Now think of things in your life. What is so bad after all? It is indeed a beautiful life. It is all about you, for you, through you, as you, with you. There is a Chinese saying: "You will see the vastness of the sea and the emptiness of the sky if you just step back one step; you will gain calmness of mind and harmony of *qi* when you yield three inches." It is not always about being right that is important. It is about being happy, healthy, and having the quality of life that matters. Chinese Daoism also emphasizes the importance of choosing harmony, happiness, and peace over being right or wrong.

The way you perceive things determines your reality. Life is supposed to be the soul's journey. Heavily conditioned as we are, we tend to think the worst of ourselves, asking too much of ourselves, perceiving things from this non-supporting perspective. It is essential we learn to unwrap gifts in the here and now and enjoy the bounty of life. This by itself takes a shift in perspective to appreciate.

I once looked at my distribution business as being beneath me. Coming from ego identity, I remember thinking to myself years back, "For heaven's sake, I was a college teacher back in China. Now I am delivering merchandise to stores for resale in America," and felt sorry for myself. When my college roommate came to visit me in America, I took her with me when I visited my distribution customers. It was so amazing that she competed with me to carry the basket I used to move merchandise to the stores, saying that it was her free weightlifting exercise. Then in a follow-up letter she sent to me once she was back in China, she stated that what I did was really beneficial, making money while having free exercise every day. She further elaborated that because it was a way of life, I was automatically exercising my muscles without trying. I didn't need to use my spare time to exercise purposefully as other people had to do.

Wow! That opened my eyes to the business I had built from scratch, realizing it was not bad at all. In fact, it was very good. So now in the whole scheme of my life as an author, a holistic health practitioner, and a YOUNG MIND YOUNG BODY transformational health coach, I look at that part of my life as my fitness program. In a real way, it is beautiful! I visit friends who have supported my family and me for over a decade through our consistent business relationships. It helps put food on our table and a roof over our heads. It also offers me insight into being an entrepreneur in America, experiencing the taste of running a small business wearing many different hats – purchasing, serving customers, employee training, overseeing resources, sweeping floors, cleaning the toilet, and so on. It has gifted me the real-life experiences I would never have learned from the MBA program I attended on the East Coast.

In retrospect, I see that it is exactly what I need to fulfill my soul's wish for the next chapter of my life, spreading my rippling effect of wellness and wakefulness in the world that is sleeping in chaos and disharmony.

How can you harness the power of perspective to your advantage?

- **First of all, observe your perspective on things**. Then ponder why you have that particular viewpoint. How does it serve you in life? Acknowledge your viewpoint. Understand where it comes from and what causes you to think that way. Dip deep, get intimate with yourself, and understand yourself more. For years I harbored resentment for taking care of things for everyone, shouldering the burden of the business, cooking, and cleaning. So I developed a practiced of showing this anger; you know, the loud sounds, pots and plates banging, thinking that I was doing everyone a huge service. These prolonged outbursts of frustration led to living with a man who was constantly angry and uncooperative, and my daughter was exposed to that unhappy living environment. It did not matter that I did all these things, what mattered was the manner in which I did them. After much reading, reflecting, healing in all senses, and learning more about myself, I started to look at things differently. I started to focus on my daughter's well-being and my own health, wellness, and happiness instead of insisting on getting things done a certain way while making everyone miserable, especially myself.

- **Second, shift your mindset to create a new perspective that will serve you better**. When we change the way we look at things, the things we look at change; when we change the way we are with things, the things we are with change. Consider the perspective on growth. Some people come from a place of stagnation, and settle in the comfort of misery or mediocrity. Some look at life from the perspective that change is the certainty of life, and therefore constantly stretch out of their comfort zone. Growth is the norm for them, which in turn brings out the exhilaration that comes with expanding. If you hold the idea or perspective that growth is only for young kids, stagnation settles in. Consequently you pass through life dying a little every day.

I had a taste of that in the past. I would rather live fully and be alive than let perceived security and certainty hold me down. Nelson Mandela said, "There is no passion to be found in playing small – in settling for a life that is less than the one you are capable of living."

- **Third, make mindful intentions and act on establishing new sets of perspectives that reflect your new outlook towards life.** This is life's work, and it starts with awareness. Your thoughts are very powerful. Be very mindful of how you choose your thoughts to reflect your reality. Choose your perspectives wisely. Make sure they reflect your truth rather than the conditioning and expectations of others.

- **Fourth, if something bothers you and doesn't dissolve after you give it some thoughtful digging, look at it from different viewpoints.** Maybe you can view it from the place of a sage you love, the author of a book that resonates with you, someone you respect, a historical figure, maybe even a stranger on the street, maybe that homeless person you saw the other day. What would they each say about it?

8. Ride the Waves of Life's Challenges

The Chinese word 危机, meaning danger, consists of two words: crisis and opportunities. It means opportunities lie in danger and dangerous situations create opportunities. We are facing one of the most challenging of times in history. On the physical plane, the whole world economy is crashing down, especially in America. Tons of homes have been foreclosed on, and many homes are sitting idle due to job loss and a sluggish economy. A large number of people have lost or are losing what they worked for their whole lives. Accompanying this outward melting down are the chaos, disharmony, illness, crimes, wars, anger, and hatred that originate from people walking away from self, from each other, and from the whole.

It is also the best of times. There have never been so many opportunities in the history of mankind. There is so much to be done – epidemics of disease, low energy vibrations, and the disconnection with source. The world could literally be reshaped! And the seeds are literally within! There are so many people waking up from the inside. They have been rising above circumstantial challenges, coming out of hiding, and answering the calls of our times. They're becoming health coaches, holistic healers, life coaches, and motivational leaders at a time when we need healers and educators the most. They are consciously raising the total energy vibration, waking up the sleeping public, and helping with transcending our lives as a whole.

On a personal front, most of us have more challenges than ever with home economics, personal health and wellness, relationships, and, most important of all, the unsettling anger, resentment, frustration, complaints, stress, and no direction. On the other hand, these are the perfect circumstances to wake us up, forcing us to come to the realization that these are all mind-induced creations of our own. If we could only shift our consciousness, our true reality is ours to claim, where happiness is a matter of a choice. Life might seem challenging from the conditioned point of view, but these challenges can be met with nothing more than showing up for our evolution.

You are a soul residing in the field of unlimited potential and possibilities. You are a spark of that universal life force, expressing that universe (uni-verse: one song) in your unique way. You chose a physical body that came equipped with the ability to experience pain, pleasure, desire, security, fear, anger, frustration, fatigue, depression, and a heightened sense of being. This very act sets you up for challenges in life. On the one hand, if you were to sail through life blockage-free without any barriers, you wouldn't feel any real sense of accomplishment or you wouldn't be challenged enough to get down on your knees, asking the whys, and suddenly come to the realization that life is simply to be treasured and savored in the here and now. On the other hand, when physical pain and the many associated sufferings are too much to bear, they might make you sick, which damages the physical house that is your body, and then you won't be in a position to fully enjoy the fruits of life.

I have heard so many times that everything you have ever wanted is just out of your comfort zone. By stretching, you are tapping into your essential nature of unlimited potential and possibility. This is the key to unleashing the mass of creation and experiencing the sensation of exhilaration and bliss, which is the purpose of your soul's journey. Your life, by your own soul's design, is filled with challenges that you can find the inner strength and resources to walk through and come out more resilient. Once you understand challenges and crises for what they are, you can adjust the way you look at these barriers in your life and view them as something to guide your way back home instead of having been sent against you. They are here for your evolution, for unresolved issues to be sought out in this lifetime, and to open up certain channels to wake you up to certain lessons and wisdom.

Knowing this, you can calmly face challenges as they come, focusing all your energies on the solutions instead of getting angry and frustrated. I witnessed my own emotional display with the challenges in my life. It was as if the universe was testing how far I could stretch without really getting me so sick that nothing could be reversed. The lessons needed to be loud and clear enough for me to reset my direction and get back on track from the detour.

In early to mid-2000, I got involved in real estate investment. With the compounded variables of bad tenants; costs of lawsuits, maintaining the properties, and high and rising property taxes; and the real estate market crashing down, I was presented with the real challenge of losing all I had worked for. I let the stress and fear of the possibility of losing everything material get to me. It caused me to worry constantly. I pressured myself to make more money to save a situation not worth saving. Consequently I was stressed-out about paying for properties that only brought me stress, misery, and hardship. So this stress showed up on me as unshed body weight that refused to leave me for years. Of course, nothing happens in isolation. Everything in our lives is so intertwined and closely linked that one thing leads to another, a vicious cycle, until you learn to break the pattern by waking up from the inside. I intuitively know that everything happens for a reason, but what was the reason here? I found myself asking the question over and over: "Why me?" For a while I found myself asking, "Why not me?"

In retrospect, I knew my soul was sending me a message, telling me that I was off course and that the detour of running after money and a false security was far too long and far too deep. So I was being presented with the financial challenge as well as the emotional and physical ones, to wake me up to realign with my center and get in touch with the person and the life I was destined to live. My healing journey has been a process, just like everything else is in life. It is designed to be this way so we can all assimilate life's experiences in our own ways, at our own pace, in the eternal here and now.

It might seem that you are facing the crushing down of the life you built. But rest assured that it is just a process of things falling into their proper places, following your inner growth, as if your life is being reorganized to reflect the new, real you. You won't be faced with these challenges if you are not equipped to dance through them. The universe has you covered. The daily practice of getting in touch with the source residing within you powers you up in living through the storms while you are thoroughly savoring every moment of it.

One day a friend of mine sent me a scripture passage about David shepherding sheep, drinking in the peace, serenity, and beauty of his surroundings. It hit me with the strong and clear revelation that the real meaning of life is to be totally absorbed in the here and now, connect with the Divine within and all around, and be one with the universe regardless of where you are and what you are doing. True, you might be presented with challenges in all areas of life. Regardless of how huge or gigantic these challenges are, they dissolve and become nothing under constant conscious and intense presence. On top of that, they become your path and a part of life, just as easy as cooking, walking, meditating, staring into a lover's eyes, or playing with kids. When you live life that way, that child inside you comes alive.

It all boils down to how you view life's challenges. Here is how I have been learning to make challenges in my life work for me instead of running me down:

- **Silently observe and witness**. Every time you face a crisis, calm down, find your center, and observe yourself from there with no judgment. Are you reacting to the situation or responding to it? What are you feeling and where in your body do you feel that feeling? Then ask yourself what the solution should be. If it is urgent and you don't have much time to sit on it, go with your gut intuition and live with the decision. Normally, when you are observing yourself in action, the decision or response naturally comes from that place of totality. The universe supports you in your decisions synchronistically once you have made them. If you have some time on your side to sit on the decision for a little while, do exactly that. Find some solitude, maybe during meditation before you drop into that stillness in between thoughts. Ask for guidance with a solution. Then move on with life as usual, trusting that the answer to your quest will be delivered to you in the form of insight, thought, or someone who shows up as the solution. Resist the urge to come up with a solution by thinking until your head hurts. By practicing this way of being, you will find enjoyment, songs, rhythms, magic, and the beauty of life.

I remember a few winters ago, I was driving on the highway in my Sprinter truck that I use for deliveries, and a dash light came on, indicating an oil shortage. I was at the end of a very bad case of the flu that wouldn't go away, and I was not feeling so well. I got off the highway and drove to a gas station. Of course they did not have the oil I needed because it is a diesel truck. In the process and commotion of opening and closing the hood, the latching mechanism of the hood got damaged. *Now what?* I asked myself. Not only did I have an insufficient oil indicator on, now the hood would not close. I could just call my road service provider and have them tow the truck back to the warehouse or to a shop and have the problems fixed later. All along I had been observing myself from the calm center, finding myself responding and accepting the situation as is. Somehow deep down I knew everything would be taken care of.

So instead of getting hysterical, I just stood by the hood and looked around, and right next to the gas station was an auto repair shop. Long story short, they were not experts in my kind of truck, but the owner knew enough and was kind enough to buy a few quarts of diesel oil tailored for my truck. It was personally delivered to his shop within the hour by one of his local suppliers, charged to me at his cost, and he put the oil in my truck as a courtesy. While waiting for the diesel oil, he had one of his guys in the shop straighten out the hood latch and put it back on again. I was back in business!

When I thanked him with a choked voice and a heart full of gratitude, he was almost choking himself, so happy he was able to help me out. I can still remember his wonderful Texas accent ordering oil for me and calling me a *gal.* My trip home was a very emotional one, full of gratitude, inspiration, and the resolve to spread my rippling effect in transforming lives. This story will stay with me forever. In this case, my crisis was the window for me to experience that beautiful humanity, compassion, love, and caring for others, and the sense of unity, oneness, and togetherness. I would not have felt it so profoundly and deeply if I had not been in that pinch, with a high fever and shivers, and icy snow all around, needing a solution.

- **Learn to embrace uncertainties**. At the most basic level, everything is particles bouncing around randomly that shape the nature of our world as constant change on the backdrop of stillness and non-change. This makes our lives unpredictable. It can be a very good thing if you look at it in the sense that it helps keep your life unfolding, enabling you to tap into more of your potential, stretch your muscles more, and grow more resilience. It is the wisdom of unpredictability that keeps fresh blood coming and prevents life from becoming stale and stagnant, leading to decay and death. In the past, like most people, I had trouble living at peace with uncertainties. I have been getting better at embracing uncertainties in life by consciously learning to live life through the center. That fear of uncertainty mainly drove my struggle in the past, trying to build up something for my old age. I was driven to create the certainty that my physical body would be taken care of in my later years at the cost of getting sick in the here and now. I sacrificed living to chase a perceived future security, and ended up not having any certainties besides the certainty of being sick and miserable.

YOUNG MIND YOUNG BODY is a delicate dance and a fine balance of the physical, spiritual, mental, and emotional to reach and gain the totality of true living and being the beings we are. You don't want to sacrifice one at the cost of another. The wisdom of uncertainties is to keep change constant, blood circulating, creation spurring, and the life force pumping. This is the way everything around us operates, including our own bodies with their cells constantly renewing. Biology tells us that within a year's time we have a brand new body. The only reason we can still recognize a friend not seen for years is pattern recognition – the formation within the similar pattern. This is the best news ever, offering us endless potential and opportunity to shape our bodies the way we dream they can be, making them the best extension of our soul's desire and the embodiment of our essence.

- **Drop the words *try* and *trying*; just get at it**. *Try* and *trying* is a mentality. It means that you must put forth an effort to get something done and that life is a struggle. The reality is that you either do or you do not. Trying is a useless mental struggle. In trying, you are working yourself up to doing something you avoid doing. A person can get tired by trying, and end up doing nothing. Next time you catch yourself trying, simply drop that mind-induced useless exercise and get at the things that need to be done. Take that email you have been trying to write – simply write it. Once done, it is over, period. The email campaign you've been trying to launch – schedule a time for it and launch it according to plan. Small tasks can become challenging and daunting if they are not being kept up. We often use the word *try* to postpone things that we never really intend to do. Again, observe yourself without judging when you say that you will try, or you are trying. Understand it for what it is and get it over with. If it is an excuse for something you hate doing, now you know the answer. If it is just a habit, learn to switch it into the actual doing.

9. Simplify and Downsize

I often wonder how I have managed to get myself into all this clutter and stuff. All I ever really need is a roof over my head, a good bed to sleep in, a functional kitchen to cook in with nourishing and wholesome raw foods, and some clean, clutter-free space to live well – basically a nice house and a moderate income sufficient to meet my basic needs with some for wants and rainy days. This is easy to accomplish without adding stress. But instead I had been blindly chasing after some sort of misguided security, driving myself to the point of breaking down to accumulate houses and stuff. The irony is that the more I wanted to accumulate to cling to that sense of security built on material accumulation, the less I was able to keep it, and saw it go down the drain with the housing market crash. That opened the door for me to see the true reality of things, the unpredictability, the ambiguity, the constant change, and the impossibility of a happy life based on material accumulation.

There is nothing wrong with material things that serve you. The truly important thing is whether you have aligned yourself in ways that ignite the spark of life within you, allow you to use your special gifts and talents that you have come equipped with for the universal message to come through, and sustain you while benefiting the world at large. If you have, you are truly living.

I have heard it said many times that when basic needs are met, with some means for wants and security, it promotes flourishing and a sense of abundance. Anything beyond that, and unhappiness and stress start to set in.

When I was growing up, when we had enough food on the table and some extra money to buy clothing, we were all happy. Many of us get into the trap of wanting more, spending money we have not even made to impress friends we don't even like to show that we have it made. Then we keep at it, fearing that if we don't we will be perceived as less than what we are. The truth is, we are struggling and bleeding internally and externally, working for something we could live comfortably without. It might look hilarious from the viewpoint of an onlooker, but that's what most of us do, day in and day out.

It is time to go back to the basics, downsize, and let go of a way of life that no longer supports you as the person you are. Years of doing and accumulating can also take years of undoing and decluttering. Letting go does take time, resources, and conscious intention, especially the intention that accompanies deep transformation. Look at it as part of life and lessons to be learned. Be patient and be gentle with yourself and others in this process. Blaming is not going to solve anything, besides adding stress and damage. Focus on where you want to see yourself. Hold that vision steady and fast in your mind's eye, and build around that. Don't get sidetracked by anything while hunkering down in the here and now, living in awareness. Here are a few suggestions:

- **Live your life for yourself, not for show**. Anything you do, anything you buy, is for your benefit only. It is something that can address your needs and wants, and your family's, based on your budget and lifestyle. Let it be something you can easily integrate into your big picture. For example, when making the decision to buy a house you have to factor in location, size, style, payment plan, taxes, your preferences, tastes, lifestyle, whether it's in the city or country, large or small, cozy or spacious. It should be easy to afford without adding much stress or affecting the quality of life and health for you and your family. Keep in mind the friends you might be unconsciously trying to impress with your new purchase whom you don't even like and are not the ones who are going to pay your mortgage – you are. That certain image you are trying to keep up does not mean beans in the end.

- **Spend some time pondering, reflecting, communing with nature, or simply being.** Cut down on some of the busyness that results from constantly being on the go, driving kids to all sorts of activities, and attending gatherings – especially the ones you really hate to attend but are afraid not to because of being judged as the odd bird or being unsociable. Sometimes "fitting out" is just as necessary as fitting in. In the end, it really doesn't matter whether you are there or not if all you do is try to keep up boring conversations or tolerate meaningless chats.

- **Be very cautious of impulse buying.** The best thing is to have a budget and only use cash instead of charging to your credit card. Once I started being conscious about my buying behavior, I caught myself buying on impulse quite a bit. It was very surprising, because I always thought of myself as being frugal when it came to family economics. Somehow over the years I got into that behavior without even knowing it. No wonder I found so many duplicated, unnecessary, and useless things in the house. I was not sure what to do with them. They simply sat there accumulating dust, cluttering space, and draining energy. True enough, in my family I was not the only contributor to that jungle of mess. I was just not aware of what I wanted and was influenced by that habit without making conscious choices of my own.

- **Spend a little time each week picking through the items that have been bothering you the most**. Put them into two piles, one for things you might need – some might even be in the original packaging; the other for things you don't need or want. Unpack items that are still in their packaging, and if you want to keep them, put them in the appropriate places; have them serve you right away. Repair and put to use broken items that mean something special to you. Hold a yard sale to get rid of some things. The best thing to do after the yard sale is to drop off everything that wasn't sold at a collection center or donate it to a charity. You might even get a tax write-off. You can make it into a leisurely activity if you are interested in flea marketing. You could enjoy the warm sunshine, lazily chatting with people coming by while getting a little something for your "junk." You could also test-drive eBay. This exercise does not need to be overwhelming; you can just take baby steps. But you have to start somewhere. A neat and orderly house will be reward enough, serving as your rejuvenation center.

Live your life from a place of ease and simplicity without the excessive burden and material overkill. Simply strip away all that is unnecessary and get down to the basics where life is uncomplicated, simple, light, and stress-free.

Chapter Three

Meditate into Your New Reality

1. Spirituality

It is impossible to talk about meditation without touching upon spirituality. It is the life blood and essence of YOUNG MIND YOUNG BODY. From where I am now, it is unimaginable to live, be myself, talk, and write without coming from a deep place within. That is where I consciously operate from now as a being living wholesomely, simply, and truthfully.

We are beings who can live to be whatever we can dream of being, without limitations and boundaries, and even go far above and beyond our wildest of dreams. There is a force out there that makes things go round; life continues, with death as a natural part of the circle. That force originates from a vast emptiness and nothingness that holds the potentials and possibilities for everything imaginable and unimaginable. That unmanifested vast nothingness is simply space. It is the source where everything originates and the place to which everything eventually returns. It is timeless, shapeless, spaceless, ageless, and non-local. The nothingness resides in stillness, and eternity is love when it moves.

The consciousness or soul of each and every one of us resides in that nothingness where thoughts cannot reach. We all draw from that endless, bottomless, universal oneness, and constantly feed back to it with everything we do or do not do in the form of energy vibrations. Our consciousness is all-knowing. Our awareness of that innate knowing is what waking up is all about. To get in touch with that deep knowing is to tap into the eternal, unlimited source that is never born and will never die, and to get to know the grandness, magnificence, and perfection that we are as beings.

Spirituality is all about getting in touch with our true reality while we are in our physical bodies in the here and now, experiencing life so that we can come to the knowing that we had it perfect all along. We need to come to that knowing through life's experiences, regardless of what they are, until bliss – that innate, natural, permanent orgasm – dawns as our reality. The best part is you don't need to fight for that eternal sensation of bliss to become your reality. The contrary is true: by simply "allowing" and letting go, you are in that state of joy where you laugh for no reason and smile because your nature comes through you. Just be – you will be on top of the world, in your bubble of highs. That by no means says that you sit idle and do nothing. It is a state of being. You can go about living the dynamic, versatile, and powerful life of a hurricane and stay calm and peaceful in its eye.

The way we perceive things, feel things, experience life, and assimilate those experiences is fed to our individual subconsciouses as imprints. It is through constant observation in awareness that those imprints are brought to the conscious level. That consciousness does not exist in our bodies. The famous neurosurgeon Wilder Penfield looked for the "record" of decision-making in the brain, but he could not find it. This suggests the possibility of something beyond the brain, like the human spirit. So where is it?

It is understood now that it exists in that nothingness. It is a space where there are no thoughts – that is in between thoughts and beyond the thinking mind. It is a space where particles are flying around randomly. In quantum physics, it is called *Brownian motion*, or "*poll of mush*," where anything ever being dreamed of can happen. Some call this great place God, some call it Divine, some call it Providence, and there are other names for it as well. In China it is called Dao (道).

A few have mastered the art of merging this physical reality with that divine force which we all have access to. We have Jesus in the Western world; Rumi; Muhammad, the messenger of God, in the Islamic religion; Gautam Buddha in India; Zen in Japan; and GuanYin and LaoZi in China. Many more have reached this enlightened god-state of being but have chosen to remain silent. What else do the enlightened need to say when they are in that space of stillness and silence where they find their bliss but remain silent so they won't be laughed at or misunderstood by those who have not experienced that? I am so very grateful that many enlightened ones have chosen to talk and write about this blissful sensation they reach. We all have this God-nature within us waiting for us to discover and connect with.

I grew up in a time in China barren of religion, when the only option for worship was Mao ZeTong. There was a song that went, "When the sun rises, the east becomes red, Mao Ze Dong appears in China." Mao was elevated to sun status, whereas in the physical plane he was the very symbol of ego at peak expansion. Under Mao's leadership, a thousand years of traditional Chinese culture – historical figures, tales, and many other cultural inheritances – were treated like garbage to be disposed of and removed from people's consciousness and subconsciousness. That time period was called the Chinese Cultural Revolution. So naturally I grew up with no knowledge, following, or understanding of any religion. I did inherit of a rich culture and insight into the way of things and the natural order of the universe simply by being surrounded by people who were the natural carriers and bearers of that culture, even under the extreme circumstances. Politics could never really take this culture away, which is in the blood and being of its very people.

When I came to America, I was approached, lectured, and pursued by many people from different religions. The intriguing thing was that the principles of all the religions were similar, teaching people to be good and to treat others with love, tolerance, respect, and understanding. The people who were preaching to me all showed the common traits of passion, love, faith, and admiration when they told me about the glories of God in their religion and about their religion being the best, the only one to redeem a person from his or her sin. Then there was the display of disgust on their faces, in their voices, and in the manner in which they spoke when it came to other religions, not to mention the common conviction that all other religions should be forbidden like forbidden fruits.

I was confused, to say the least. Many people told me that I needed to have a leap of faith – to just believe in the God they believed in and stay away from the others. Then I would be saved after I died. I did not know which one to believe and didn't feel right in my gut to believe in any. But all the while I knew there was a force behind everything. It was only when I was on my healing journey years ago that I was again pulled towards spirituality. This time it was through my reading of Deepak Chopra's work. It finally hit me: We all share the same GOD, the same source. It is because of physical, geographical, and cultural differences that we have different god figures in our various cultures. Now that makes perfect sense to me.

Our God has to bear our way of living, like everything else in our lives such as food, clothing, traditions, etc. So naturally, with the emergence of cultures, traditions, and countries resulting from the movement of people throughout history and the separation of regions by geographical topography, our God moves with us as well. God is molded into the life we are familiar with. Even our ideas of heaven bear the things we appreciate and want more of in this physical life, and the idea of hell is a fire burning in eternity.

If every one of us could soak up the essence of love in the oneness of this cosmos and allow it to be the guide to everyday mundane living, then when the sense of oneness and everyday living merge in sync, we ourselves could become as enlightened. In actuality, we are all divine beings, with the universal God living and expressing through our unique signatures.

My first yoga and meditation teacher said something to the effect that enlightenment can be reached by many means, whichever works for you. Believing in a certain god figure can help in reaching that state where the inner and outer merge and the gaps in between thoughts become longer and longer until you are one with all there is. You truly become the conduit of the universe with no thoughts, just impulses and messages. You are enlightened. You have become the truth.

Spirituality applies some of the same ideals as in religion, but it imposes no borders and no limitations, and it opens to everyone and everything. The essence inspires us all to live freely, happily, and in exhilaration, peace, and harmony. God, it seems to me, doesn't have a religion, but an omnipresent presence of love assists us in creating a life of free will while, in the process, unleashing our divine essence from within.

2. Benefits of Meditation

Meditation is quite a buzzword these days, and the practice is popular in all walks of life. The media talks about it. Tons of books have been published on the topic listing the benefits of this traditional Eastern wisdom, and many people meditate on a daily basis. Many leading experts in the rising alternative healing field have been spreading the practice of meditation as well.

I heard Dr. Andrew Weil, director of the Program in Integrative Medicine at the University of Arizona, talk about the calming effect of one particular breathing technique he practices on a daily basis. And I heard him say at IIN that meditation is one of the best low-cost, low-tech alternative medicines, assisting in disease prevention and aiding in our bodies' built-in healing mechanisms. Deepak Chopra, in partnership with Oprah Winfrey, has led many twenty-one-day global online meditation challenges.

Meditation's range of focus is wide in the world of healing, anywhere from perfect health, happiness, joy, and abundance to revealing destiny and impacting the world on a very large scale. In my Transformational Author Experience program with Christine Kloser, she always started the sessions with a guided meditation, helping everyone get centered and present.

On one of my daily walks with my daughter, we went to a bridge to listen to the water running and watch the trees. As we stood over the river, the idea hit me to do a short thirty-count deep-breathing exercise with my then eleven-year-old daughter. This "One Minute Meditation" was taught by one of my IIN Ayurveda (an East Indian healing modality) teachers, Dr. John Douillard. I knew this practice would help tremendously with her attention span and the surprisingly large amount of stress she was experiencing from peers, homework, and school in general.

I told her to follow my lead, breathe in deeply all the way to the belly, then breathe out and let go of all the stale air, for thirty counts. We remained absolutely quiet and still for a few minutes in that profound peace and calmness, and then we opened our eyes. My daughter was so surprised at the heightened sense of beauty opening up in front of her. She told me that the leaves were so green that they were almost blue to her. She said everything was so much more pleasant and pleasing – birds singing, water running, crickets chirping, the wind rustling – all were singing the songs of nature's beauty and life's rhythm.

It was one of those occasions when my daughter wanted to walk more, constantly talking in a very cheery manner. It was also the time she told me I was beautiful. I needed to have more confidence in accepting that truth about me. We have made the thirty-count deep-breathing meditation part of our walking routine whenever we make our way to the bridge. It has never failed to induce that "wow" effect from my daughter. I even practiced the thirty-count deep-breathing meditation with some of my neighbors over by the bridge, and all experienced heightened calmness and a peaceful sensation. There is a reason people are meditating and connecting outer with inner, physical with spiritual, and source with extension.

I have meditated regularly since the beginning of October of 2011, at the beginning for about ten to fifteen minutes per day, then I increased it to about thirty minutes per sitting, two sittings daily, one in the morning right after getting up and the other before bedtime at night, with many impulsive meditations in between. I am a new person. I am still emerging, with constant ahas!, new insights, new delights, and new heights. I am able to carry that deep, peaceful, meditative state of mind throughout the mundane living of each day. I am full of creative ideas and naturally high most of the time. My baseline energy vibration stays peaceful, tranquil, and relaxed at times when I am pulled down by the forces around me. It provides constant support for my health and vitality.

I am grateful that I am creating my own reality with conscious choice-making in here-and-now awareness. I am grateful that I am able to live life from the center. I am grateful to walk the talk of healing the world doing what I love to do – speaking, writing, living, and coaching. I am grateful for my regained robust health and rekindled young mind and body. I am enjoying my life as it comes, whatever way it comes, and I am in NO HURRY to rush it. I am just following the flow.

Granted, there are bumps along the way. At times I have been challenged to the core, not knowing what to do and what to think. Then again, I learn not to think. I simply take a deep breath, get centered, stay grounded, and listen to the guidance from that place of totality within.

At times I also incorporate deep breathing and meditation in my coaching practice to bring myself, as well as my client, fully present in the here and now – to create that sacred space of healing where my client feels safe, at ease, and willing to be vulnerable and exposed. This is the place where true healing begins.

When you close your eyes and go deep into that quiet place, you have gone where there is no beginning, no ending, no time, and no space. It is a place where you are never born and will never die. It is a place where you can recharge your life force. This magical place is within every one of us. It is when you tap into that unlimited potential and embrace your uncertainties that true transformation starts to happen.

Meditation is by far the best way to go to that space. You might feel the calming effect the first time, or it might take you a bit longer, depending on the quality and duration of your effort. The first few times might stir up some disturbance; just as when you clean house there is some dust floating around at first, and then it starts to settle down. Once the layers and layers of conditioning and blockage have been penetrated, you start to truly reconnect with your source. After a while you might find yourself approaching life's challenges or everyday hassles with a calmness you never before knew you possessed.

You might start to look at everything as itself instead of through the emotional factors involved. You might even be able to look at your emotional traumas and patterns from a distance. You might not be offended as easily. You might view things from a more neutral point of view. That puts a glow on your face and vibrancy in your being, drawing more smiles and looks your way, even from strangers. You might find yourself saying "My day is great" when being asked how your day is. You might find love bubbling in your heart, saying "I love you" to everyone, causing some surprises and wrong perceptions from the deeply conditioned world. These are by-products of being deeply immersed in that permanence – the unity, the oneness, the togetherness, and the inseparable stage where we are as cosmic beings.

In the quantum world of swirly energy, there are no clear boundaries where one thing ends and the other starts. In a very real sense, you are part of me and I am part of you, with the basic interaction being energy waves. Our emotions, thoughts, and feelings intertwine and influence one another through the waves of energy. With the practice of connecting with your center through meditation by going inward, you might also find yourself filled with sympathy, empathy, and compassion. You might be able to feel the pain, joy, happiness, and uplifting energy from those around you. You might want to help others who are suffering or need a bit of uplifting.

You might feel this profound gratitude, heightened joy, and swell for being alive. You might find a profound quietness within you as well. The floating dust, noise, contradictions, and complications might start to ease off. You might start to compare yourself to others less and live your life for yourself instead of always seeking approval from others.

You might also start living a life of simplicity, since simplicity is our essence. You might start looking at things from the obvious, instead of overcomplicating things. A friend of mine said it best: "When you are simple, your world will become simple." You will be able to gain clarity, focusing only on things that matter and letting go of the rest.

It is a lifelong process. Many of the complications in the physical realm reflect the buildup of inner complications. Let it be okay that it takes a while, maybe years, for simplicity to register on the physical plane while you are peeling through layers of conditioning and shedding redundancy in the here and now. Intensely engage in this process with full awareness. I feel I can do anything I set out to do, as long as it makes my heart sing. You can have that, too. All it takes is just learning to connect with your energy and happy source. With time, you will be able to feel the miracles of life. Your experience might be different from mine and others. Profound peacefulness, calmness, and restfulness seem to be the common denominator.

I often wonder why everyone is not jumping on the meditation wagon. It is free and takes no investment of any kind other than time. It has no known risk of any side effect, except maybe being calmer, happier, and more vibrant and ecstatic, plus even looking years younger. Or maybe I do know, from my own past, why people are not meditating into a new and better reality. It is because most of us are too buried in our perceived world, worrying about stuff and rushing through life without truly living. We come to think that is how life is – struggling, worrying, and fighting battles, with some occasional laughs and giggles mixed in. We can all relate to that. To make it stick, I list below in further detail some of the documented benefits so that you'll know that it is for good reason that this Eastern tradition has been followed for thousands of years and embraced by millions in the world. Once you get the knack of it, you will want to kiss happiness and joy fully on the lips.

Now you have an idea what meditation can contribute to your health and well-being. I could say that anytime you see someone in their forties, fifties, sixties, even seventies who is peaceful, vibrant, and youthful-looking with fire and love in their eyes, chances are they are deeply connected with the inner through meditating or another way of getting in touch within. You might be ready to get started without bothering with reading more about the benefits of meditation below. You have my blessings, and I will meet up with you in that space of formless, shapeless, timeless, ageless, where everything originates. If you happen to be someone who won't do anything until you exhaust all research, then read on. If it is not enough to nudge you to meditate, you will have to dig deeper yourself, but I highly recommend you start meditating while you dig so that the added dimension of experiencing it firsthand, instead of simply taking in the knowledge intellectually, will make your searching more meaningful. It is the actual being in that space beyond the thinking mind that makes the difference in you and your life.

Countless studies have been done to validate this Eastern wisdom of connecting with the source through meditation. You can Google "benefits of meditation," and a long list of research will come up stating various physical benefits. So far I have not found anything negative other than the advice to not attempt meditation if your mental health is poor. Modern scientific techniques such as MRI and EEG have been applied to monitor what happens in the bodies of meditators and how their bodies and brains change after meditating regularly. *Buddha's Brain,* written by Dr. Rick Hanson, a neuroscientist and researcher, shares many of the current scientific research and investigations in meditation, with the main conclusion that positive emotions such as love can be strengthened through meditation. Hanson's viewpoint represents a popular movement to study and embrace Eastern wisdom and practice, including meditation, in the Western world.

- **Benefiting the brain:** During the latter twentieth century, collaborative research in neuroscience, psychology, and neurobiology focused on meditation and its impact on brain activity and the central nervous system. It sought to define and characterize various practices. The impact of meditation on the brain has been categorized into two areas: state changes and trait changes. State changes reflect the changes or alterations in brain activities during meditation, while trait changes are the accumulated effects of a long-term meditation practice. All the findings direct us to the understanding that a person is more relaxed, while remaining aware, in a meditative state. Long-term daily meditators also experience brain-state changes in higher-order executive and associative cortices. This supports the Eastern knowing that meditation increases self-regulation and attentiveness.

- **Increased love and compassion:** Dr. Richard Davidson, a world-renowned psychologist and author of *The Emotional Life of Your Brain,* a *New York Times* bestseller, wrote about changes in the brain observed when comparing before and after brain scans of a group of people who went through two weeks of love and compassion meditation training, half an hour per day, totaling seven hours. They behaved more altruistically. It looks like any amount of meditation practiced on a daily basis can remap your brain in the right direction. Due to the plasticity of neurons in the human brain over its natural lifespan, it can be influenced by the outlook a person takes on life regarding everything they see, think, and are exposed to. Your brain can change, for better or for worse. The good news is that you can train your brain to be happier, sharper, and calmer.

- **Reduced need for sleep:** A research study by Prashant Kaul, Jason Passafiume, R. Craig Sargent, and Bruce F. O'Hara titled "Meditation Acutely Improves Psychomotor Vigilance, and May Decrease Sleep Need" published in *Behavioral and Brain Functions* in 2010 suggested that meditation may be able to replace a portion of sleep such that six hours of sleep plus two hours of meditation produce the benefits of eight hours of sleep (in addition, of course, to other benefits from the meditation). My introductory meditation teacher told me the same thing when I told her years ago that I was feeling tired and needed more sleep. She said something to the effect that if I were to meditate I would need less sleep and feel more energetic, more alert, and more in my element. I find myself telling friends, clients, and even strangers to meditate if they cannot sleep. I find it much easier to wake up naturally in the morning, at about the same time each day, ever since I started practicing meditation daily. Falling asleep is much easier as well. And the quality of my sleep has become so much better over time.

- **Calming effect:** Our nervous system, as mentioned earlier in chapter two, consists of a parasympathetic system and a sympathetic system. The parasympathetic system regulates heart rate, breathing, and other involuntary (automatic, or without our realizing we are doing it) motor functions. The sympathetic system gets us into the fight or flight response by releasing the stress hormone. Meditation reduces stress and increases relaxation.

- **Therapeutic use:** Meditation is practiced in mainstream health care as a stress-reduction and pain-reduction method. It is used by hospital professionals in cases of chronic or terminal illness to reduce complications associated with decreased immunity caused by stress. The medical community agrees that mind-induced stress leads to declining physical health. There are more research projects planned and underway to further study the benefits of mindfulness practices such as the various kinds of meditation.

- **Prolonged and heightened awareness:** Mindful practice, wherein a person trains the brain to pay attention to breathing, an image, or a beautiful feeling such as happiness, love, compassion, or holding a light, flame, or glow in the heart or third eye (in the middle of forehead), is intended to increase attention span and ignite insight. A prolonged and more flexible attention span makes it possible to be in the here and now – to be aware of a situation and be able to observe from a distance and obtain a creative awareness of flow. It becomes far easier to apply emotional intelligence in emotionally or morally challenging situations. Countless findings suggest that in a meditative state a person is more relaxed while maintaining sharp awareness.

- **Slowing down of respiration:** According to research from Harvard Medical School ("Functional Brain Mapping of the Relaxation Response and Meditation"), physiological signals show that during meditation there is a decrease in respiration and an increase in heart rate and blood oxygen saturation levels.

- **Aging benefit:** The 2009 Nobel Prize winners for biology, Dr. Elizabeth Blackburn and her colleagues, found a correlation between stress, the length of the telomeres (a structure at the end of chromosomes that protects chromosomes), and telomerase, an enzyme that protects chromosomal caps from the wear and tear of cellular division and aging. The more telomerase we have, the longer our telomeres will be; the less telomerase we have, the shorter our telomeres will be; the shorter our telomeres, the more exposed we are to aging, degeneration, and disease. It is concluded that mindful meditation might decrease stress arousal and directly increase a positive arousal state. Increased telomerase activity promotes longer telomeres, possibly leading to cell longevity.

3. Let's Meditate!

To begin, find a quiet place. Sit down with your legs crossed, or stretched out in front of you if you feel your legs are too stiff. With your palms up, mentally let go. Close your eyes and breathe in and out slowly and deeply through your nostrils, thinking of nothing. If a thought occurs, simply watch it go with the out breath and keep breathing in and out. If it helps, direct your attention to your breathing. The gap in between thoughts is the magic space you want to fall into, *dropping into the gap*. True meditation builds an intimate connection with yourself by going deep inside. Outside influences such as music, sound, chanting, or guiding words are not necessary, though these can be helpful in quieting down that busy mind in the beginning.

It might take some time to quiet down your mind. Should you have any disturbance or unsettling feeling in the beginning, stay with it and give it time and space. You might start to feel the calming of the mind and a sense of relaxation right away. After a while, you will look forward to that moment of peace and rejuvenation. Do it every day. Start with five to ten minutes and shoot for thirty minutes – not as a rule, but as a simple guideline for a daily routine. If you have a knack for getting up on the wrong side of the bed in the morning, it's a great way to help you get out of the habit. We have all known people who are grouchy in the morning, and would do anything to stay away from them at that time. I still remember greeting a coworker I had years back with "Good morning" each day, and he would mumble something like "What's so good about it!?"

Train your mind to hold one image. Pick something nice, supporting, beautiful, and loving, such as a sunset, a beach with seagulls, the image of your lovely pet, your

ing face, a beautiful picture, the perfect moon peace and tranquility, or the morning's rising light, energy, and promises. You can picture yourself rising up with the in-breath and falling down with the out-breath. Should you find your mind traveling all over the map, dwelling in the past and racing into the future – dinners to cook, things on your to-do list, bills to pay, phone calls to make, places to go – simply bring your mind back to that single image or thought.

You can also start your meditation by imagining yourself sitting under a big golden arch or inside a golden circle. You are protected. No harm can hurt you or reach you. The arch beams a wave of gold. Take that in for a few minutes. Then start acknowledging your body, from head to toe, mentally making sure each part is okay. Start at the top of your head, where the sixth chakra is. Then your hair, the skin of your head, both your ears, your forehead, eyebrows, eyes, under the eyes, nose, cheeks, upper lip, lower lip, tongue, upper pallet, lower pallet, throat, and all sides of your neck. Then move to your shoulders, upper arms, elbows, lower arms, wrists, hands, and all your fingers from your little fingers to your thumbs. Then your back, to your spine, and to the front of your body, your chest, and belly. Move down to your thighs, upper legs, knees, lower legs, ankles, the soles of your feet, and your toenails, from your big toes to your little pinkies. Take your time doing this. You have nowhere to go, nothing to do, but sit here idly appreciating your body. Once you are done inventorying the parts of your body, thank them for being there and doing their parts to make your dream of experiencing sensual experiences possible and allowing you to fulfill the destiny of realizing your perfection by design – the goodness, the wholeness, the oneness, the love, and the timelessness.

You can practice the short thirty-count deep-breathing meditation all the way in and out of your root chakra where your basic life energy – sex energy – lies, in and out through your nose, and then be still and quiet for as long as you would like or time permits. Open your eyes slowly afterward and look at the things in front of you anew, as if you zoomed in with a sharper lens. Your senses might be more heightened. Things might appear to be shapelier, more pronounced, more colorful, and fresher. The quick thirty-count mediation does not leave room for any thoughts to come in, which places you in the gap where everything originates, to recharge, rejuvenate, and restore.

The other technique you can use to get you in the flow of peace, quietness, and calmness, with very few thoughts in between, is to focus on one object your eye can see, be it a beautiful picture on the wall or a candle flame. Keep staring at it with all your attention until your eyes want to close. Then just close your eyes without fighting it. Put your attention and focus in between your third eye, which is at the center of your forehead, and your two eyes, looking for something, but with no particular expectations. Don't let it be something you have conjured up in your head. Just be there, observing, in your wakeful awareness.

Another approach is to look at an envisioned flame in the third eye area. Some suggest looking at a mental vision of a flame in your heart area to hold your attention. If music is what gets you to quiet down in the beginning, by all means put on some soft, soulful music of your preference. Let your attention follow the flow of music, reaching down to your heart and soul.

You can also follow a *guided meditation* to get past your mind to that meditative state. In the process, you will be training your brain to quiet down. There are tons of YouTube guided meditations. For starters, you can look up Deepak Chopra, and there are many others. Listening to soulful, chanting music is a favorite of mine to get into that space of ancient wisdom where my soul is calling to me. One chanting meditation that comes to mind is from Deva Premal and Miten. You can listen to their guiding mantra meditation on YouTube. See firsthand if it resonates with you. You can then go from there and get more for your collection of aids for your daily meditation practice, or simply do your own thing, you and yourself, the old-fashioned way. With eyes closed, simply sink into the sound of permanent stillness.

Once you quiet down, sounds seem more pronounced than usual. When you go beyond that, you are with your essence. I do love to feel the sound of stillness and allow it to carry me to its depth, wrapping me inside its magic and healing power. Sometimes I feel slightly dizzy from the swirl of energy and sound, which reminds me of the sound of circadian rhythm. Often it is when you are looking for stillness that you notice all the sounds. If you are in a quiet place, away from modern-day noises, you will hear the sound of nature, such as the rustling of tree leaves, birds singing, crickets chirping, your own breathing, your heart beating, and the sound of stillness and timelessness. Once you get into the thoughtless space, all disappears but your essence.

Depending on your mood, whether you have rested well, how depleted your body is, how restored you are, and how deeply connected you are, you might see images. Be with it. Be open to it. It could simply be that your soul is telling you something. You might simply fall asleep, which happens quite often in my before-bedtime meditation. This is okay because meditation turns on your parasympathetic system dominance. It enables your body to relax. So whatever your body needs at the time, it will show up during meditation. Go with your body's natural instinct. Give it what it needs. Once your homeostasis is balanced, you won't be falling asleep. You will stay aware and calm. This is a good benefit of meditation before bedtime, promoting quality sleep.

Sometimes I wake up during the night and cannot fall back to sleep right away. Knowing I need the rest to function at optimum the next day, I just sit up straight in a meditating position, take my mind to that peaceful rejuvenation center, restore, and rest. In most cases it brings me to a sleeping state very quickly. In cases when the sleeping state is not reached in short order, I just remain in that leisurely state of mind to recharge without pressure or stress. You might feel heaviness or lightness in your limbs at times. That's all good.

Meditation does require you be healthy enough to sit up with your spine straight, enabling the flow of energy, or *qi*, to go through your spine and throughout your whole body, moving oxygen to your brain. If you have a physical issue such as a weak spine, injured back, hurting shoulder, or neck ache, you might want to address it while getting your meditation practice started. Yoga is one way to address a physical issue. The stretches were specifically designed for a person to be flexible enough to meditate to the state of enlightenment where the union of body, mind, heart, and soul takes place. Yoga stretches can not only train your brain to be calmer and facilitate the opening up of subtle energy channels for energy to rise to the crown chakra, but also loosen up some of the tense muscles in your body, promote the growth of new pathways, stimulate the growth of new cells, and serve as a maintenance measure for your body for sustaining stability, strength, and flexibility.

I read a research study, collaborated on internationally, that was sent to me by the Zen group. It said that by just sitting idle, letting your mind wander and roam free, you can reap the benefit of increased creativity and more calmness. It goes to say you will benefit even if you can't quiet down the noisy, busy, thinking mind in short order.

Once your mind quiets down, true meditation is simply getting in touch with self with no outside distractions and nothing in between. That gap you experience where there are no thoughts is when you are one with your consciousness, or soul, or the universe, or Divine, or Providence, or God. Whatever you want to name it, it is the source of creativity, oneness, unity, love, and light. The longer you meditate, the better chance you will get into that gap without thought occurring. A life lived this way is very transformational and rewarding. It might not look like much of anything, sitting there for ten minutes to half an hour on a daily basis, maybe two sittings per day, but it adds up. The key is to keep up with the practice and loving self-care. Don't expect miracles to happen or to be enlightened the next day. The practice in itself by itself is very healing, relaxing, and rejuvenating. Simply enjoy the journey.

Some days you might have better experiences than others, when you experience profound peace, tranquility, and flow of insight. Other days you might feel dry, falling off your high, pulled down by everyday living and the people in it. Let it all be okay. That's how it is. Just keep at it. Sooner or later you will find yourself looking at everything and everyone, every chance meeting, every happening, from a much calmer center. You might get used to observing yourself from a distance, being able to forgive and understand. Your focus might shift to what really counts in your life.

I would like to share a story about what happened to me one day, and the responses, the thoughts, and the feelings I had, which I wrote about in a blog post. I shortened and edited it here:

> How Would You Feel If You Were Me?
>
> Last Friday, at about two thirty in the afternoon, when I came out of a gas station in Chicago to my parked car, I could not make sense out of what I was seeing: shattered glass all over the driver's seat and the passenger seat. Then I saw the passenger side window all broken, with shards left around the edges. Suddenly it hit me. Someone just broke my window and stole my purse! In it, I had everything to establish me as a normal everyday person: my phone with access to everything, my credit cards, driver's license, many other cards, keys to several places, and about one thousand dollars in cash. For quite a few minutes, I just stood there and stared at the scene. I did not know what to think or feel. Then my mind started to move. Oh my gosh! What am I going to do!? Then I went over to the passenger side to confirm that the window had been broken on

purpose, by someone who took my purse that had been sitting in between the two seats while I was making a quick trip to the gas station.

The next thing I remember is that I quickly walked into the store and told my long-term customer there that my car had been broken into. He rushed out with me, checked the situation, then went back to the store and started to view the video. It showed that when I pulled into the parking lot in the front, another silver van pulled onto the side street. I stayed in the car for quite a while, probably checking my emails. As soon as I locked the car and walked into the store, a medium-built young Mexican-looking man wearing a cap with the visor pulled low walked towards the passenger side of my car while talking on his phone. He looked in and then walked away. Still on the phone, he walked back again and broke my window. Then he was off the phone; both hands were holding something in the front. Obviously, the object held was my yellow, fringed, India-style purse.

With the help of my friends in the store, I walked around to the back side of the store, thinking that he might have just taken the cash and left all the documents and personal items somewhere, maybe in the garbage container. Then I went through the motions of filing a report with non-emergency police using the phone at the store, contacting the credit card companies to cancel the stolen cards, and asking my phone company to disconnect my number from that phone and disallow my number from being registered with any other carriers.

On the drive home through Chicago afternoon traffic, I found myself asking questions. "Why me?" Then "Why not me?" "What is it trying to show me?" "What does it say about me?" "Why do certain people always want something from me?" Then the thought occurred to me, "Just maybe this guy needed that money so much more than I did, so much that he was willing to go through the fear and act of breaking my window, leaving me the mess to deal with." Another thought came up just as quickly: "The son of a bitch is just being plain lazy, doing drugs or something, having no concerns for others or who he is hurting. He is so much in his own world of misery that he never thinks of others, unaware of the consequences of his actions."

In the process of establishing the normalcies of my life, I have met so many good people I am grateful for. The strangers in the store showered me with sympathy; the customer service people; the police taking the report. Three Will County police officers showed up at my door just wanting to make sure we were safe, constantly reminding us to call if we saw anything unusual. The very young officer told me not to lose hope in people as a whole because of one incident. Steger Police dispatched more patrol to my warehouse location, making sure no one who had no business there would mess around Friday night before we had the means to change the locks and secure the location.

I could be miserable, resenting the man who broke my window and stole my purse, not seeing the kindness, compassion, support, and love from my fellow humans. I could write this off as a bad experience. Instead, during the whole time, I had been observing my own feelings, emotions, actions, my spoken and unspoken words, my thoughts, the food I ate, and my other self-care routines. And to my delight I found myself remaining in my center, not getting overly excited about this whole thing, besides the cracking up of my voice saying, "I feel like crying," and a few sobs, releasing some of the old conditioning of unworthiness, and a few times calling my purse stealer "lazy."

When I was waiting for my car window glass to get installed, I was reading Panache Desai's book, *Discovering Your Soul Signature*, about anger, shame, guilt, and all the other unworthiness feelings resulting from fear and insecurity. I was also reflecting in the direction that we as beings are one in essence. It's our separation from ourselves and each other that causes us to feel this feeling of shame, inadequacy, lack, greed, anger, and frustration, and that was precisely what had happened here. It was an act most of us would associate with shame. It was something not to be proud of, something to be condemned, similar to some of the shame we are carrying around in ourselves. The truth is that we are all in this together, waved in the universal pool of consciousness. We influence one another with our waves of energy, in the form of thoughts, feelings, emotions, actions, and state of being. In the sense that everyone who appears in our life is for our benefit, this guy who took my purse, without telling me of his intentions, in the most fundamental way is my brother, a part of me, and is for my benefit. It is a fact hard to digest. If I were to truly love myself, how could I resent or condemn him without doing the same to myself in an already not-so-pleasing circumstance?

The thing that came to mind most was the challenge we all face. How to be healthy, vital, and happy despite life's happenings. The fact that no police were being dispatched to investigate a crime like this one is a very common thing, happening often. My thoughts linger on all the challenges we seem to face on a daily basis, on the different scenario of how I would be reacting if I hadn't had about three years of deep connecting with myself, day in, day out, aligning with inner and responding from this calmness that only true source can provide. I could imagine myself being angry, as I did in the past, adding a few years overnight. So in the end, I marveled again at the wisdom and power of the source we all share and have free access to. I felt the profound gratitude for waking up to the wisdom of applying self-love and self-care in my daily life, to keep the house of my soul in perfect condition to experience life as it comes, in whatever form or shape it comes, with no distinction between good or bad.

To make it more interesting, before the theft I had just been talking with one of my clients about the transformational journey I had been on. How I looked at everything in my daily life on the physical plane from a calmer center. How I did not play the drama queen role any longer. How I saw things for what they were. At the time the stealing episode happened, my mind went back to the conversation I had had with that friend just one hour earlier, wondering about the coincidence of things. What was it teaching me here? Just when I had been talking about facing life's challenges with peace and calm, I was being tested in such a way. The following week I went back to her store and told her about the incident, which of course invited the unavoidable question of whether that was a real challenge. She smiled and nodded her head, saying, "You are okay, seeing you laughing telling the sorry tale."

Connecting with true source does have its everyday practical implications. One of my yoga teachers told me in a private conversation that when you had meditated long and been with the source long and deeply enough, you would feel the Divine doing your daily chore for you, through you. You would not feel the pain of mind-induced physical stress. When there is no thought occurring, organic creation spurs forward, pouring out. In a true sense, you start seeing yourself and seeing the world around you from a different place.

True connection happens when you are not in the thinking mind or when you are in a "no-mind zone" with only pure awareness. Many of the Zen masters from Japan reached enlightenment through sword fighting and archery. It is a state where you are not trying through thinking hard, but relaxed to a point that you allow the universal power to carry out your intention through you, and the response from you is organic, totally from your center. A good way to understand this is to imagine that your house is on fire. You would want to run out and avoid being burned; there is no time for thinking because you have to respond quickly to stay alive. I have been reflecting on ways to incorporate this organic, total, non-partial response in my life, with everything I do, to live and create the life I want for myself.

Given that, in anything you do, as long as you are in the here and now in that physical body of yours, you can achieve the no-mind zone. Many of the Daoist qigong masters have obtained "the way" by practicing mind-directed, graceful, slow movements mingled with stillness. Meditation can happen practically anywhere, anytime. It can be while dishwashing, when the warm water runs through your hands while you watch birds flying and singing outside your window on your blooming crabapple tree. It can be walking in nature when you are absorbed in the lushness of greens, harmony, and the peace of nature. It can be simply sitting in your backyard where the sun warms your body while the gentle wind rustles through tree leaves, caressing your face and soothing your being. Or it can be dancing on ice, relaxing into the rhythm and flow.

The pure joy of being has its texture, color, shape, path, and even scent. It differs for everyone. I cannot tell you how yours will be. You will have to experience that for yourself by actually meditating. It is really worth the time spent. In the end, you will be so glad you made meditation part of your daily routine.

Start meditating. Experience for yourself the pure joy of being. With this heightened sense of joy, life will be different. You will create a new reality for yourself out of nothing. You will start to look at things from a different place – a place of abundance, gratitude, ease, and alignment. Don't just take my word. See it for yourself.

Chapter Four

Live in Harmony with Your Surroundings

1. You Are Part of a Harmonious Cosmic Whole

Nature's cycles are determined and influenced by the positioning of the sun and moon. Nature dominates everything in our daily lives. We are part of nature and the height of its evolution on the physical plane. It is essential for us to follow the clues and lessons from nature, with all that entails. Ancient cultures have long since related human life, health, and healing to universal life and the cycles of nature, and have been proven to work wonders for thousands of years in both the Eastern and Western parts of the world. There is a strong, growing interest and trend to combine these time-tested healing modalities with modern, up-to-date technology and science.

The Chinese Five Elements theory, linked with the philosophy of yin-yang (阴阳) balance, has been developed over thousands of years. Evolved over time, it has been perfected by everyday practice, from planting to deciding on dates for marriages, locations for houses, dates for building houses, and the medical use of applications in wellness promotion and maintenance. According to this theory and way of life, when everything is in perfect sync, man with nature and nature with man, things go with ease, grace, and natural flow. When things are out of harmony and balance, disease forms and develops and over time becomes something major and affects the quality of life.

Five Elements principles say the cosmic world consists of five major elements: water, wood, fire, earth, and metal. Everything in this world is made of the same elements, from the faraway stars to the mountaintops, trees, animals, bushes, flowers, houses, and the human body. All things in the cosmic world are intricately intertwined, closely linked, with one influencing another, either promoting, restraining, or even destroying. A good healthy life is to gain harmony among the elements, dancing within the opposite polar forces, harnessing balance and harvesting from the destructive natures of the elements. These Five Elements in nature have internal regenerating correlations, but also destructive and restraining natures. It goes something like this:

> **Generating interactions:** Wood feeds Fire, a campfire for example; Fire burns woods to become Earth (ashes); Earth bears Metal, like the gold you might find in your backyard; Metal makes Water more beneficial, due to the mineral content; and Water nourishes the growth of Wood.
>
> **Overcoming or destructive interactions:** Metal cuts Wood, like using an axe to cut wood for your fireplace;

Wood entrenches Earth, such as roots reaching deep down into the earth; Fire melts Metal; Earth absorbs Water, which is why earthly dirt has been used to build water dams; and Water puts out Fire, which explains the fire hydrants in front of houses.

Restraining interactions: Fire evaporates Water, such as in home cooking water evaporates into the air after reaching the boiling point in a pot, or the sun dries up small bodies of water; Water washes Earth away, in the cases where water volume is large enough to wash away a small volume of earth dirt; Earth (rock) destroys Wood; Wood dulls Metal, which explains why an axe needs to be sharpened after being used to chop wood for a while; and Metal shields against Fire.

The same Five Elements are also associated with the phases described in nature, including humans, as five phases: Wood/spring – period of growth, abundance of woods and vitality; Fire/summer – swelling, flowering, brimming with fire and energy; Earth/late summer – fruition; Metal/autumn – harvesting and collecting; and Water/winter – stillness and restoration. Each of the phases takes seventy-two days. Further correlations are stated below, summarized by my going through much online research in addition to my readings; my natural heritage of being born and reared in the countryside in China, picking medicinal herbs as a child, starting out in life being a very sick child often treated by a Chinese medical doctor and by a mother who was constantly boiling Chinese medicinal herbs; attending Chinese medicine classes; and talking and learning with my Chinese doctor friends.

I introduce the Five Elements in detail below not to confuse, but to provide a glimpse into the intricacy of connectedness that all beings and forces in nature share. This doesn't even scratch the surface of the vast knowledge of the Five Elements and Chinese medicine. Take note that the correlations were obtained throughout Chinese history by observations and practical everyday applications. The concept of *association* is important in understanding the various aspects of the Five Elements. To avoid the repetition of using the word *association* and the *is* and *are* statements every time, I omit them altogether by using a dash, as in "body part – tendons" in the description of the wood element instead of "the body part for the wood element is associated with tendons."

> **Wood**: The materials associated with wood elements are wind, sound, plywood, air, minerals, acid, mind, rubber, paper, static, wax, health; the color is green; the shape is rectangular; the cardinal direction is east; the planet is Jupiter; the heavenly creature is the azure dragon; the phase is new yang; the direction and natural phenomena are expansive and exterior and in all directions; the season is spring; the climate is windy; the sprouting is in developmental growth; the mental qualities are idealism, spontaneity, curiosity; the emotion is anger; the internal organ, or *zang*, is the liver, a yin organ, the inside organ of the pair; while the yang organ, or *fu*, is the gall bladder; the sensory organs are the eyes; the body part – tendons; body fluid – tears; finger – the index finger; sense – sight; taste – sour; smell – rancid; life – birth time; and animal – scaly.

By these descriptive associations alone, you can pretty much tell when your wood element is out of balance; you will have liver or gall bladder issues, may develop poor sight and teary eyes in spring, and things will taste sour. When in balance, you will be emotionally happy, feeling expansive and full of hope. A person with a strong wood element is very goal-oriented, sharp, ambitious, and good at planning and executing.

Fire is associated with the planet Mars and the mental quality of passion and intensity; emotion – happiness; *zang* (yin organ, or inside organ of the pair) – heart or pericardium; *fu* (yang organ, or outside organ of the pair) – small intestine/San Jiao; sensory organ – tongue; body part – pulse; body fluid – sweat; finger – middle finger; sense – speech; taste – bitter; smell – scorched; life – youth; and animal – feathered.

When this element is in balance, a person is full of fire and energy and has good digestion and robust health. When fire is out of balance, it shows up as inflammation, overheating, heart problems, and mouth sores. The person is very vulnerable in hot weather. Bitter-tasting foods like leafy greens can help balance some of the imbalances, bringing the person back to the balanced state of fire. Walking can help restore the balance as well.

Earth is correlated with the planet Saturn; mental quality – agreeableness, honesty; emotion – love;

zang (yin organ, or inside organ of the pair) – spleen/pancreas; *fu* (yang organ, or outside organ of the pair) – stomach; sensory organ – mouth; body part – muscle; body fluid – saliva; finger – thumb; sense – taste; taste – sweet; smell – fragrant; life – adulthood; and animal – human.

Earth people, when in balance, are the most grounded, patient, caring, nurturing, and peace-loving people you can have around. They are easygoing and pleasant to be with. When out of balance, they tend to meddle in other's affairs, gain weight easily, and love sweets, and their bodies tend to make excessive mucus. The best thing to do is to gain the groundedness again by eating more root vegetables, warm foods, and sweet vegetables to satisfy the natural sweet tooth. Earth people flourish in late summer, the Indian summer.

Metal correlates with Venus. It is linked with the mental qualities of intuition, rationality, and mind; it is associated with the emotion of grief, sadness; *zang* (yin organ, or inside organ of the pair) – lung; *fu* (yang organ, or outside organ of the pair) – large intestine; it has not been assigned a sensory organ; body part – skin; body fluid – mucus; finger – ring finger; sense – smell; taste – pungent; smell – rotten; life – middle age; animal – white tiger; and color – white.

Well-balanced metal people are intuitive, rational, and well organized, and work well with set rules. They thrive in the fall when the temperature is cool and colors are vibrant. They breathe better at this time of year. When out of balance, metal people tend to be grief-stricken and lost in sadness. They might be overly critical, be prone to lung-associated breathing problems, and suffer from frequent colds, maybe asthma. They might develop rashes since the lung meridian rules the skin.

Water corresponds to Mercury. It has the mental quality of erudition, resourcefulness, and wit; emotions – fear and scare; *zang* (yin organ, or inside organ of the pair) – kidney; *fu* (yang organ, or outside organ of the pair) – urinary bladder; sensory organ – ears; body part – bones; body fluid – urine; finger – little finger; sense – hearing; taste – salt; smell – putrid; life – death; and animal – shelled sea life.

The characteristic of a water person is very determined; they can overcome hardships by sheer will power, and succeed in their pursuit. When the water element is balanced, a person can be fearless, forging ahead. When out of balance, a person may start to be fearful, indecisive, anxious, and withdrawn. A woman weak in the water element during menopause displays the symptoms of heat and dryness, showing up as hot flashes, night sweats, dry skin, and dry throat. Kidney yang weakness is associated with cold extremities – cold back, cold belly, declining sexual vigor, and increased urinary frequency or incontinence.

All of the five internal pairs of organs are assigned a time period as well, which helps doctors and patients determine the best times to take different medicines tailored specifically for different organs, but I won't cover that, as my intention is to show you how closely linked we are with nature, as one. I talk a little more about the time aspect in later chapters about sleeping and bodily movement.

Ayurveda: I was exposed to Ayurveda over the years in working closely with my distribution business customers, of which an overwhelming majority are from India. Most have substantial knowledge bearing the inheritance of the Ayurveda life philosophy and medical wisdom. At IIN, Dr. John Douillard, one of my favorite guest teachers, brought Ayurveda as a life philosophy and medical tradition to a new light. This enabled me to further grasp the intricate and intertwined relationship we humans share with nature and our environment. As with the Chinese Five Elements theory, Ayurveda breaks the seasons into three predominant seasons – spring, summer, and winter – and the corresponding body and personality types, or *doshas,* into kapha, pitta, and vata. The seasons and dosha types share similar characteristics, strengths, imbalances, anecdotes, and stages of life, reinforcing the truth that we humans are part of a whole. To be healthy and vibrant and nourished by nature, we need to live by nature's laws and cycles.

In spring, it's most beneficial to eat what is growing naturally outside, such as leafy greens and berries, to cleanse and break down the excess fat accumulated over the winter and get it out of the system, similar to the Jenny Craig diet that is so popular these days. When spring rolls into summer, more fruits and vegetables mature into the building, cooling, nourishing foods with high carbohydrate content that sustain the beings we are during the longer days and hot weather. In late summer there are more apples, maybe even pomegranates, available to assist us in ridding ourselves of the excessive heat buildup from summer days, through loose bowel movements. This gets the body ready for winter by reducing the likelihood of a cold virus settling in through the dry conditions caused by excessive heat left in the body. When summer progresses into cold winter days, people living off the land become dormant, staying indoors and living off the rich harvest of the fall, such as all varieties of root vegetables, through the methods of fermentation, preservation, and cooler storage. They consume more building and warming foods, such as soups and stews, fats, and meats, in the right portions, of course. These foods help them survive the harsh and cold winter elements through more body heat and insulation layers in addition to wearing more warm and heavy clothing.

Kapha, or spring, is the season of childhood, a time of growth, a time full of mud and mucus and wet conditions. Mucus-inducing foods such as pizza, large quantities of cheese, and meaty products further feed this unhealthy and imbalanced trend. Instead, a more balanced food group with more cleansing and clean, building qualities is more in alignment with this growth period, especially for a growing kid in springtime with a kapha tendency. When in sync with nature, this growth period is very spongy, active, and healthy. It bears the quality of springtime, with upward growth.

Pitta, or summer, is the season of adulthood, with strong heat and a fierce, burning life force. Everything is going strong, steady, and productive when in balance. With the steady progression of early summer to late summer, human bodies experience a similar type of growth pattern, from rapid growth to maturity. To be healthy and vibrant, overheated conditions need to be watched out for. Imagine an overheated, inflamed athlete running a marathon on a hot summer day in hot, dry Las Vegas, eating hot and spicy food! He is going to be inflamed and on fire. So the ability to slow down, the habit of eating cooling foods, and practices such as qigong, yoga, and meditation all help bring an overly heated pitta person back into balance with the highly productive, healthy, and vibrant state of being. It is an intricate dance to maintain the right amount of fire: inspiring, energetic, firing enough, yet without the downside of overheating, causing inflammation and damage to the body resulting in early aging, fatigue, and burnout in a pitta-dominant person.

Vata, or wintertime, is predominately air quality and dryness. It is also the late stage of life when the life force is spent. Experiences have been accumulated over a lifetime of living. More wisdom is gained. A person is wiser, more philosophical, and airier. He or she is not much into material things anymore, and instead more into spiritual growth and intellect. To bring this person into balance, into a more grounded, warm, and solid state, warm grounding foods such as root vegetables and stews are beneficial. The diet from the health-food movement is good, too. To understand the type better, imagine a cold person in cold, windy Chicago in the cold winter eating raw, cold foods; all I can think of is one thing: COLD, and I find myself shivering just imagining it.

With the Ayurveda philosophy of living in alignment with nature, we would naturally be one with self, merging physical with spiritual, in union with nature, in unity with one another, and in tune with oneness. It is the original and natural order and nature of things. It is where our true essence of love, kindness, happiness, vitality, timelessness, agelessness, and bliss dominates. It is where we are at peace with ourselves, with our surroundings, and with the people around us. It is where life is no longer a struggle, but bliss lived in sync with everything and everyone around, creating, loving, and living to explore one's full natural potential.

Greek medicine: I often heard about Hippocrates being the father of modern-day Western medicine, the four humors, and Greek medicine. I was naturally very interested in taking a look at how the original form of modern-day medicine really worked and what it really was about. To my surprise and delight, I found more things that support my findings about how living in alignment with nature keeps one peaceful and healthy. As a traditional holistic healing system, Greek medicine has a lot in common with Chinese medicine and Ayurveda. These traditional medical systems seek to harmonize the health of the individual with the universal life forces of nature and the cosmos. Like Ayurveda, Greek medicine is humorally and constitutionally based. Like Chinese medicine, Greek medicine seeks balance, or homeostasis, between opposite yet complementary forces of nature, according to Greek Medicine.net, established by David Osborn, master herbalist, astrologer, holistic health consultant, and educator.

The Greek tradition views healing as the gift of God. The first gift was a goddess named Gaia, mother earth, the source of all nurturing, growing, supplying, sustaining, and healing in accordance with mother-earth principles. Later on, the Gaia hypothesis was formulated by James Lovelock as one global healing consciousness governing all living things. Everything interacts, co-depends, corresponds, and communicates with the environment in which we live. The entire planet is creating, supporting, nurturing all lives, healing, and maintaining health on planet Earth. For all living things, being in harmony and peace with the surrounding environment means surviving, thriving, reproducing, and multiplying, while violating the rules means suffering, sickness, disease, diminishment, and death. In this sense, nature and healing medicine are considered a coherent ecosystem, with one feeding the other and affecting the other, and one change calls for a chain of changes, for better or for worse. Like Chinese medicine and Ayurveda, Greek medicine also relates the human body to the natural elements. The four natural elements in Greek medicine correspond with the four humors that are the metabolic agents of the four elements in the human body – phlegm, blood, yellow bile, and black bile; and the four seasons, the stages of life, the time of day, and personal characteristics.

According to Greek cultural philosophy and medicine, the cosmos is made up of the four cosmic elements in varying degrees: earth, water, air, and fire. Earth is the solid state, the center, as the ground we walk on, the planet whereon we dwell. Because of earth's groundedness and heaviness, everything else gravitates towards it. Around this planet is water in the form of rivers; oceans; lakes; other waterways surrounding the earth, connecting earth, and giving living things life and growth; and the rains pouring down onto earth, nourishing or flooding the earth. Air, representing movement, contact, and exchange, is everywhere above and around the sphere of earth and water, giving living things life through breathing. Finally, fire is the force for transformation. It's the force that lights up the sun, the moon, and the stars. It's also the life force living through everything, including humans. The four elements that make up the cosmic world also make up human bodies and body parts, in varying proportions and composition:

Water – Phlegm – Winter – Phlegmatic: The water element corresponds with the phlegm humor and the season of winter. It is cold or cool, and wet in temperament, according to Greek medicine. This causes the phlegmy condition, fertile ground for the cold virus to take root, so a cough, nasal congestion, running nose, tearing eyes, and other cold symptoms show up more often. It is also the stage of old age, frail and cold in body temperature. It corresponds with midnight of the twenty-four-hour sun wheel, from 9:00pm to 3:00am. A phlegmatic person holds much phlegm in their body, is rarely emotional, and is more rational in responding to things.

Air – Blood – Spring – Sanguine: The air element relates to the blood humor and the growing season of spring. It is the temperament of wet and hot or moist and warm, where everything is in the upward sprouting and growing season. New life comes forward with rapid growth. Tree sap, the essence of trees, rises up to the tree tops, bringing life back to the trees and green and growth back to nature. The human body is more alive with quality exuberant blood. Spring fever captures these phenomena quite accurately. It is also childhood in the stage of life, where growth, expansiveness, sponginess, and aliveness are the key characteristics we see in youth. Spring is assigned the hours of sunrise, from 3:00am to 9:00am according to the six-hour quarter of the Greek medical chart. A sanguine person looks radiant, healthy, and rosy, and bubbles with happiness and youthful vitality

Fire – Yellow Bile – Summer – Choleric: The natural element of spark and life force, fire is associated with the humor yellow bile, the season of summer, and the choleric constitution. It carries the temperament of hot and dry, where moisture content evaporates with the rising heat. The hot, dry condition irritates yellow bile, leaving humans feeling feverish and agitated. This characteristic corresponds with adulthood – with choleric drives and ambition – full of vigor, energy, and plans to move forward with life, yet impatient, irritated, and agitated when out of balance. In the twenty-four-hour circadian cycle, fire is the six-hour time period surrounding noon, from 9:00am to 3:00pm, when the sun is most direct, intense, and hot.

Earth – Black Bile – Autumn – Melancholic: The natural element of earth is associated with black bile in the human body, the season of autumn, and the constitutional type of melancholic characteristics. In fall the weather cools off, but the dryness stays. It makes fall cold and dry, which aggravates black bile. This season relates to the afternoon of the circadian cycle, ranging from 3:00pm to 9:00pm, rendering it somewhat melancholic, gloomy, cold, and dry. A person at this stage enters middle age, an age suddenly seeming to be very close to old age. One might suddenly realize the shortness of physical life and the many unfulfilled

> dreams, wishes, and yearnings, leaving one feeling the passing-through and melancholy of life. For many, awakening dawns at this stage of life as well. This is the time when so many middle-aged people start to slow down. They might start to ponder the real meaning of life, getting on to life's purpose, and beginning the journey home to oneness, union, and togetherness. A melancholic type of person is grounded, solid, and centered to a point of being lethargic and pessimistic when out of balance, seeing only the hardships of life instead of the lightness and spiritual side of things.

The descriptions of these elements demonstrate the deep connection between the macro cosmos and the micro cosmos, a perfect mirroring of nature and the human body. The best life lived – happy, healthy, fulfilling, and living up to one's natural potential – is a life in sync with one's natural environment. Even modern-day biology reinforces this point.

To gain a deep understanding of the makings of our bodies and our relationships with our living environment, I took a college course at a local university that used the textbook *Campbell Biology*. I saw the natural evolution, the innate connection, the oneness as a whole system being demonstrated thoroughly in the college course, especially through zoom-in pictures of the biosphere: the land, waters, jungles, animals, trees, rocks, and humans, and the intricate interactions and chain influences where one change sets off a whole chain of influences while one feeds the next. I have seen the energy flow in an ecosystem – chemistry and life, water and life – and all these elements both in nature and within the human body. I have seen how everything adapts to its environment to sustain its life and how the whole ecosystem works together with organisms interacting with other organisms and the physical environment. I have seen the cycling of chemical nutrients, where leaves fall to the ground and are decomposed by organisms that return minerals to the soil. I have seen water and minerals in the soil taken up by a tree through its roots, while its leaves absorb light energy from the sun, take in carbon dioxide from the air, and release oxygen. Animals, including humans, eat leaves and fruits from the trees and take in the released oxygen from living organisms.

Energy flows from sunlight to producers (trees, plants) to consumers. Trees and plants absorb light energy and transform it into chemical energy; and chemical energy in food is transferred from plants to consumers. Consumers use energy to do work, through the mechanism of the muscle cells converting chemical energy from food into kinetic energy, the energy of motion. When energy is used to do work, some energy is converted into thermal energy, which is lost as heat. A plant's cells use chemical energy to do work such as growing new leaves.

I remember reading a book about stardust. In it, scientists who recently researched the composition of the faraway stars, galaxies, and other planets ended up learning more about ourselves. We are made of the same stuff, most commonly known as the elements in the periodic table. This finding answered our quest to know what we really are. We are part of everything, made of the same stuff as the stardust.

2. Live in Harmony with Your Environment

With the division of labor and social functions, and

specialization in skill sets, many of us have gradually and unknowingly walked away from nature and separated from the very elements that nourish and build. We have fallen into lives of superficial pursuit. We have been supplied superficial foods, with plastic wrappings; flashy, bold-lettered health claims; and bright and artificial colors, dyes, and preservatives, that will stay on our shelves forever. You might think it is good that your food never goes bad. Some kids don't even know that fruits and vegetables can actually grow by themselves as long as there is seeding, soil, nourishment, sunshine, and water. To boot, many of us are cooped up in the house, sitting in front of the TV for hours on end, forgetting there is a great outdoors where the air is fresher, the oxygen is more abundant, and the sun is shinier. We not only separate ourselves from nature, but gradually from one another, and worst of all, from ourselves. Most of us spend the bulk of our time pursuing material things, working at jobs we absolutely hate, ending up tired and worn out. We hang in there only to keep up, deeply buried in our own fear, insecurity, scarcity, lack, misery, and isolation. No wonder we are a nation of sick and sicker people. It is time to reconnect with nature, with one another, and with self. It is time to become part of the harmonious cosmic whole, learning to live in sync with our surroundings.

Here are some practical everyday applications:

- Be mindful of keeping indoor temperatures moderate – comfortable, yet not extreme. This is beneficial both for your health and your wallet. In summer, keep it somewhere around 75°F during the day when it is very hot outside. I feel very appreciative every time I walk into the house and it's 80° – our indoor temperature setting in summer when the outdoor temperature is above 90°. Keep the setting around 70° at night for ease of sleep. Dress cooler, as well as using a thin sheet to cover up the belly area, or simply wear shorts, avoiding exposing the belly to the air during sleep, which can lead to bellyaches.

In winter, keep the indoor temperature around 70° – warm enough, yet not so hot as to deplete you of the moisture in your body. High winter indoor temperatures can dry up your respiratory system, inducing the secretion of mucus in response to the dry condition in your body, a fertile ground for the cold virus to take root. Around 68° at night is sufficient, assisting with sound, quality, peaceful rest. Wear a warm, comfortable robe or sweater at home during winter, and use a heavier quilt for a cozy night of sleep. I find it easier to have a good night of sleep with a cooler temperature on winter nights, snuggling tight against warm and comfortable coverings.

In spring and fall, on days that are moderate outside, turn off the air conditioning or heating. Open the windows and doors to allow the cool air in. Let the house breathe. Allow the elements in nature to nourish your body and soul. Fully enjoy nature's free air conditioning. Be conscious not to keep heating or air conditioning on all year long. I remember some of the rental property tenants we had a few years ago. When we were called to fix something, it was so hot inside I was practically feeling sick. So many resources are wasted on unnecessary heating and cooling. It would look insane if this were being observed from outer space. We waste what is freely given by nature and use the very resources we have stressed ourselves sick over to create extremes.

I worked in trade show booths in Las Vegas a few times a year over the years. It felt cold indoors both in summer and winter. Instead of leveraging nature's free air conditioning, the temperature was set very low all year round. It was very common to see people draping large, heavy shawls over their shoulders in summer. It didn't make sense.

Look at nature for clues. Utilize nature as provider and source. Use modern conveniences just as niceties to take the edge off. We are all part of nature, part of the whole, and the natural elements are part of our essential makeup at a deep, cellular level. Being in sync with nature's laws supports the body's natural ebb and flow.

- Dress in layers during cold winters. Cover your head, decreasing the amount of body heat being pulled out of the body into the thin air. Have at least two layers on your legs, too. Your body responds to the outside environment by producing chemical compounds. In cold weather, if you don't dress adequately, your body produces insulating layers right under the skin, keeping your body heat inside. While this is good on one hand, it can pull resources away from repairing and building up reserves.

- Stay outdoors more when it is pleasant outside. Do things that bring you closer to nature such as gardening, weeding, playing in the yard, mowing the grass, walking in nature or in the woods, even chatting or doing some sort of community activity.

- Eat more of what's local and in season, so that local elements absorbed from the locally grown food support you in building your body, strengthening your immunity, and increasing your baseline *qi*. I will talk a bit more about this in the food choices section.

- Bring nature to your living ewnvironment. Keep some potted plants inside for better air and a peaceful sight. Plants emit oxygen that humans breathe in and take in the carbon dioxide humans breathe out. The interaction and exchange is very beneficial – a perfect case of giving and receiving. On top of that, greenery always brings peace, growth, and tranquility. It has a calming effect on the central nervous system, eliciting parasympathetic nervous-system dominance, where life is in harmony and peace. Consequently, the food you eat can be digested better, your emotions are more energy-building, and your thoughts are more nourishing. This can add up to building youth, slowing down or halting the rapid aging process, reversing early aging, and possibly starting reverse growing.

- During warm days in the spring and summer, when the sun is rising, stand in your yard with your bare feet on the grass and your face towards the sun, taking in father sun's yang energy while absorbing mother earth's yin energy. This helps balance your yin-yang energy, building up a bodily reserve. Standing on soil without grass is okay, too. You can also expose your back so your whole yang meridian line runs to the sun to energize. Sessions of ten minutes are sufficient in either case. It is very enjoyable, too. Or you can simply strip off your shirt or wear an exposing top to reap the sun's sunshine benefit. When you employ self-care applications such as these, be fully in it and feel the sensations, the warmth, and the leisure, soaking up nature's essence.

- On sunny days in the winter, expose your blankets to the sun. Hang them on a clothesline if you have one, or simply spread them on any clean structure with the undersides towards the sun. Not only will the sunshine kill any bacteria, but it will also leave the sunshine smell on your blankets, providing you a cozy night of snugness.

- Observe and learn from nature in everyday living. See how nature unfolds and evolves in sequence, without hurrying. A dear friend of mine put it the best: Nature does not rush, yet everything gets done in due time, as it should be.

- Mindfully cultivate a harmonious relationship with yourself and those around you – at work, in your neighborhood, with your friends, and even with strangers seen on the street:

- The relationship you have with yourself is the most important relationship of all. **Again, the relationship you have with yourself is the most important relationship of all!** A good relationship with yourself ensures perfect alignment inside out and outside in. It assists you in leading an authentic life. The guidance is always your feelings, your intuitions, and the desires coming from deep within. When you are happy from within, your essence of love naturally flows out of you. You can't help but radiate that energy to those around you, drawing more of that to you out of those who are drawn to you. Constant silent observation and reflection in awareness is the doorway to cultivate that relationship. Calm acceptance of self is the very first step. Then slowly and leisurely identify and implement changes as deemed necessary.

- Once you have grown an ongoing intimate relationship with yourself, you won't seek approval from others. You know deep down that you are enough in your own right, the way you are, whatever way you are. Chances are, once you live your truth, you will respect others in living their truths. This is the best thing we can give to the world we are sharing; that is, live our truth and show the world the truth of that which we are.

- If you can't find anything supportive to say about a person or a situation, don't say anything. I am pretty sure you can find something constructive to say in any given situation if you are fully present. Again, it is always about perspectives originating from different people with different backgrounds and experiences. There is really no pure white or black or right or wrong in many situations. Understanding this helps you look for clues as to how other people view things. See the humor and the place others are coming and operating from, thus understanding them better. Often many of their traits reflect part of you as well. This helps you understand yourself better. It brings peace of mind. A natural flow of harmony surrounds your body or comes through your body, making you feel the harmony of life's symphony. No need to be right or wrong, just happy and peaceful at your core.

- Be generous with your compliments. They are free and cost you nothing, but they offer the power of healing. They bring happiness to another soul. They brighten up their day. They light up their spirit. Suddenly their day starts to turn fabulous after getting up on the wrong side of bed. This happiness bounces back to you, taking you higher and rippling further in a happiness cycle.

- Be kind to everyone who crosses your path, even those who seem annoying. There are generally two kinds of people who come to you in your life – those who help you and those who deliver a lesson or send a message. Be grateful for whatever that is. Everything in this life happens for a reason. Whoever crosses your path has come a long way in accomplishing just that, with synchronicity at work. Imagine that! The classmates you had in college, the colleagues you meet at work, your significant other, your kids, and even the smiling strangers you happen to come across… how many things had to happen simultaneously for these chance encounters, either long term or just in passing? There are miracles in just that, so be sure not to take anyone for granted. Fully engage and understand the deeper meaning and message of any encounter. All these people are here for your benefit and for your soul's further evolution.

- Give, rather than expecting to receive, and give generously. Maybe it's giving your ear to that one person who desperately needs to talk things through. Just the gift of your presence could be the reason you are where you are or what you are at that particular time. Smile brightly at someone who just catches your eye. That sunny smile might wake up the happy soul dormant in another being. Chat with a lonely person who obviously needs some human interaction. These days, with all our modern devices, communications, and technologies, we are extremely lonely at some level. Be that human touch for someone who needs it. Giving with ZERO expectations of any return is one of the best ways to promote your own happiness. Experiment and feel its magic.

- Don't always take things personally. So many people get swallowed up by all sorts of things, necessary or unnecessary. Being sympathetic, agreeable, kind, sociable, or even just nice is not the first thing on their mind. Have empathy for them – for their isolation, stress, and unhappy inner turmoil. Don't be bothered by their attitude. Wish them happiness and move on with yours. It is really not worth it to lose sleep or health over stuff like that.

- For those you hold near and dear to your heart, it is more important to be happy and harmonious than to be right and miserable. Love them up, without conditions. Keep your ego out of it when it comes to love. Don't hold back with your love. Learn from the flowers in full bloom; they give all that they have, without holding anything back, speaking the love of life. Same thing with the sun; it shines indiscriminately on everyone and everything with its radiance, even on the clouds when they are in the way. Instead of yelling at your loved ones for leaving a trail of dirty dishes, dirty laundry, or unmindful trash behind for you to clean up, give them a hug with a huge smile on your face, love in your eyes, and understanding and expansiveness in your heart. Feel grateful for their presence in your life, and ask them nicely if they could pick up after themselves. If that is too hard for you to do, sit down with them and tell them how you feel about things. Ask for their input and help. I know it is quite challenging, especially at times when you have spent a whole day working, thinking you are saving the world from self-destruction; then you walk into a house full of dirty dishes, things scattered everywhere, cat litter smelling, and dirty laundry lying on the floor. But honey attracts more flies than vinegar. Losing your temper only makes you feel worse, and everyone else around you for that matter. It is almost like you have somehow brought with you the air of righteousness, tension, unhappiness, even annoyance to your loved ones.

I am a newbie in this department, finding it much more rewarding to be and feel relaxed with no expectation attached to anything or anyone. It actually expands me, filling me with the sensation that some of the details of life do not need to be looked at seriously all the time. It comes and goes. Life is a process of never-ending unfolding. Cleanness, neatness, tidiness, and spotlessness are nice, but are not going to happen all the time because we are living people making messes all the time. Life is messy. Cooking is messy. Living is messy. Let it be okay to be messy from time to time, as long as there is some semblance of order amid the chaos. If you are like many people these days, you have experienced the misery of having turmoil in the house, knowing deep down that all the wholesome food and exercise in the world are not going to help you feel better if you have troubled relationships. They put a huge strain on your health, sense of well-being, and wellness.

o Resist the urge to gossip, exercising judgment behind someone's back. It is unproductive in many ways, the most important being that you waste your precious energy, vigor, and life force focusing on the negative side of other people, sacrificing your opportunity to journey inward, instead of looking at the good. There is always the chance that the person you badmouth will hear about it, causing unpleasant feelings and even poor, impaired relationships. My take is that the reason people gossip is that their life is too stagnant, too unchanging, or too boring.

They have to talk about someone else to flavor it up. But that is the wrong way to go about life. The right way is to find something good to say about another person when you are about to gossip. This, in the long run, reroutes the grooves in your brain, training it to think in a more constructive manner. Another way to stay away from destructive conversations is to focus on what is important to you and your own inner growth. I am pretty sure we all have tons of growing up to do. I, for one, have the feeling I am just learning to grow up at the chronological age of fifty-two.

Chapter Five

Keep Moving

"Lack of activity destroys the good condition of every human being while movement and methodical physical exercise save it and preserve it."
–Plato

I have gone back and forth for a while about what word to use to best relay my message of exercising the body for maximum healing benefit while living life with ease and grace where stress is not part of the equation. I finally decided on the word *moving* instead of *exercising,* for the reason that there is so much more to moving the body than the current concept of exercising. There is a concept out there now that distinguishes traditional exercise as *non-functional exercise* and other types of daily bodily movements as *functional exercise.* Bodily movement in this sense includes anything that moves and impacts the body on all levels, from deep down in the cells to the exterior physical look in terms of shape, weight, fitness, complexion, vitality, and flexibility.

Exercise is quite a buzzword these days. It is very loaded, conjuring up the image of a person pushing to the limit in a gym out of sheer will, with no laughter, smiles, or happiness attached. Almost everyone knows the benefit of some sort of exercise. I often hear people say, "I ate too much today; now I have to exercise it off." Exercise becomes something of a punishment for overindulging or overeating, not something to be enjoyed. I have also seen many people jamming exercise schedules into an already busy life, adding so much stress to something they don't enjoy doing but feel has to be done to be healthy.

Exercise, like everything else in life, needs to be done right with the right mindset in just the right amount to be beneficial to the body. Too much is just as bad as too little. When it's too much, especially when you don't enjoy doing it, it induces the stress hormone cortisol and the weight-triggering hormone insulin, signaling the body that life is in danger and that fat storage is needed for survival, countering much of the effort in losing weight.

Exercise is all too often associated with losing weight, but in reality it burns very few calories. So if you are thinking of losing weight by exercising without an overall comprehensive approach to a healthy way of living, you are in for a big disappointment. Even if it works for you for a while, it is almost impossible to keep it up, since it is simply a chore requiring discipline. It is the same as being on a diet, following an eating plan you know you will abandon once you lose the weight. For a diet or exercise plan to work long term, it should be incorporated into your lifestyle to be enjoyed, savored, and carried out naturally as part of normal living, without testing your will power to the limit.

Apply the Concept of Life as Workout

In Chinese, the word 活动 (movement) has two components, 活 (being alive) and 动 (moving), denoting that if one is alive, one naturally moves around, showing the life within. Movement can be in any form, in any place, or in any circumstance. Modern-day people have a tendency to sit all the time. Almost daily, most of us sit – in front of a computer working or surfing the internet, watching TV, or commuting to and from work. How much time is left for the movement of the body to keep the muscles dense and flexible, bones strong, and cells renewing? How is it going to happen? Are we just going to be frail, weak, and without an ounce of energy, vibrancy, and youthful vitality?

There are many things you can do to keep your body moving, even if you don't have time to go to the gym and exercise in blocks of time or in a formal setting. Our ancestors didn't have the concept of walking on a treadmill. They just carried on with their daily routines to survive while keeping themselves fit, healthy, and alive. When I was growing up there was no such thing as exercising at a gym. People would probably laugh at you, wasting energy and resources like a fool without doing anything useful.

Don't take me wrong; commercial facilities and equipment provide convenience and a way to exercise for many people, especially since in most facilities there are trained trainers to help you come up with proper plans and routines for endurance, strength, and flexibility. What I mean by *movement* is something effortless, involving no stress or resolution;

something you can easily do for the rest of your life. To jam an exercise schedule into an already busy life can be stressful in and of itself, which undermines the very benefit of exercising in the first place.

If you can easily find time in your schedule to go to a gym, and the idea of working out in a gym appeals to you, by all means do just that. But when the idea of going to a gym stresses you, or you hear the voice in your head say that you have to exercise at a gym to lose weight, yet it goes against your fiber and being, simply moving is better for you. It not only allows you to get all the things you need to get done taken care of but also benefits your body as a "life workout."

I have mentioned my distribution business several times before. When I carry a bucketful of merchandise into a store, I rotate the weight frequently. I consciously distribute the weight equally so all the muscles benefit from that weight, thereby increasing muscle strength, flexibility, and bone density. I apply awareness by not pushing too hard or too suddenly but gradually easing into it while stretching my muscles. When I was growing up, the villagers kept busy the whole day from sunrise to sundown meeting life's basic necessities. They were totally absorbed in things such as preparing the soil, seeding, cultivating, watering, debugging, harvesting, chopping wood, carrying water, and so on. These activities involve bending, standing, walking, stretching, and weight-bearing. The result is a naturally healthy body weight as a way of living.

Your body is designed to move, run, jump, hunt, and gather. Modern science has proven, without a shadow of a doubt, that movement and exercise build muscle tone, density, and flexibility; increase bone density; enlarge lung capacity;

elevate mood; and sharpen brain activity. Every movement affects your body, brain, and mood in positive ways, and your cells know the difference. (I will let you do the research should you wish to dig into it further.) As long as you are living, breathing, and can still move, any movement you make is beneficial in building up health and youth in terms of new growth. The earlier in the day, the better, when your body still has more resilience to start with. Start right now, if you haven't already! It is the best thing to do for yourself, those around you, and society as a whole.

How to Build Movements into Your Daily Routine

- You reap the full benefit when you are happy doing what are you doing. Holding grudges or being angry because of the things you are doing can cause a negative charge in your system, and won't do you much good in the long run. However, movement such as walking, running, or vigorously mopping the floor or mowing the lawn can work off some steam if the anger is not derived from the activities at hand. So at times when you are angry or upset, it helps calm you down if you do some physical work or simply walk. Focus all your attention on the work or activity. It sure beats yelling, screaming, and breaking dishes.

- Always look for opportunities in your routine to get some body movement in. For example, park farther from the restaurant you are going to for lunch, your workplace, or the store where you buy groceries. If you take trains, park farther away from the station and walk the distance. Whenever you can, take trains or subways to work so you can walk more. Stretch your body and move your arms and legs. Gently rotate your head while sitting at your workstation. Run up and down the stairs instead of taking the elevator. Maybe take a walk after lunch. I once heard about a receptionist who was the only one in the office who was fit and slim because she was the only one willing to fetch copies from the copier and take them to everyone's desks while others gained weight.

Life is very fair in this regard. It reminds me of the old-time royal Chinese families getting served from head to toe. The young ladies were frail, weak, and died at a very early age. Adjusting your perspective in this regard can be of great service to your body. Run up and down the stairs in your house to fetch stuff instead of letting your kids do it for you. Serve your loved ones tea or breakfast; carry it upstairs to them from time to time. Clean the house using a mop while you play music for added fun and rhythm. Sweep the floor with a manual broom, bending down to exercise flexibility. Vacuum the carpet. Mow the lawn. Garden, weed, and plant trees, all of which require constant moving, bending, and stretching, which trains the body more effectively than pure gym exercising.

The beauty of life as a workout is that you kill two birds with one stone, as the saying goes. It is especially meaningful to me because a neat, clean, and uncluttered house and a freshly-cut lawn offer me additional benefit, allowing me to feel lighter. It further reinforces the profound calmness and quietude that has become my new baseline of being. I also constantly run up and down stairs, two steps at a time; up for strength and endurance, down for weight-bearing. Where there is an intention, there is a way. Look for ways to incorporate as many movements into your daily routine as possible.

- Bear in mind that physical movement of the body is best before breakfast because it sets the rate of metabolism for the day. More movement of the body means more calories are burning without changing anything else during the day.

- Some simple muscle-strengthening moves that you can easily do right at home such as sit-ups and push-ups do not require much time but do a lot in strengthening the belly muscles and abdomen.

- Do some mind-body exercises such as yoga and qigong to increase attention span, calm the mind, and facilitate the circulation of *qi* – life's vital energy – while exercising every joint and every part of the body. This kind of movement also helps foster a stronger mind-body connection. One of my teachers once said that doing yoga is like maintaining a car. To keep it running smoothly, the maintenance needs to be kept up. Otherwise it will break down while being driven. It's the same with the body: without mindful routine maintenance, it becomes stiff, fragile, and easy to break, causing immobility and loss of freedom.

- Find other things you really enjoy doing to move your body. I have a young daughter, so I find ways to participate in her life and have fun with her, cherishing the here and now. Sometimes when we are out on walks, she is on her bike and I run after her, sneaking up on her when she is not paying attention, which usually initiates giggles, laughter, and more chasing. When she signed up for skating class, I signed up with her. I found myself loving it and the idea of being on the ice with her and learning together. Now I can actually skate, and I really enjoy it. We even participated in a skating performance in 2015. It was so much fun that we are entertaining the idea of a mother-daughter duet next time around. We are also going to sign up for swimming classes. Doing activities with her is fun, meaningful, and beneficial, and helps keep that kid in me alive and happy.

- Test-drive whatever form of movement works best for you and how much best suits your body. Having a type-A personality, I know how it feels to overly exert my physical body, leaving me not only exhausted but losing my enthusiasm for doing any exercising at all. When I was first introduced to yoga, I fell in love with it right away. I was so delighted with the relaxing and calming effect, which was so much better for my body than forcing strenuous movement on it and becoming overly tired.

Chapter Six

Live Life with Meaning and Purpose

There might be a time in your life when you suddenly feel lost, confused, and stagnant, and wonder what the point of life is. That is your being or essence speaking to you. You come here with a plan or intention to rediscover your greatness and significance and experience certain things in life. In the process, many detours and obstacles show up on your path, pushing you to the limit, forcing you to find your true essence. Over the years I have been driven by this restless energy and have forged ahead in life, changing jobs and starting businesses. There were times I felt like a walking dead person, with no life and no drive, but a shell of a beat-up body, a worn-out spirit, and the whole nine yards of modern-day diseases, which I touched on earlier in the book.

Years ago I was walking in my neighborhood with a college friend of mine. I told her about my predicament that something was profoundly missing in my life. This was after my physical body had healed. She commented, "You have it all. What is there that is missing?" Yes, on the surface, I seemed to have it all. But I was restless. Something was not quite right, and deep down I knew it. I was not being difficult and making it all up. Deepak Chopra's work had shed light on what had been bugging me all along: the lack of meaning and purpose to ignite the spark inside of me.

When I reflected on my life, I remembered the moment when my Chinese middle-school writing teacher read in front of the whole class a composition I had written. That short writing was passed on to some other local schools. Years later I was recognized as the writer of that story by many of my new classmates when we went to high school. I can remember how I felt when they said that their teachers told them to model their compositions after my writing. There was also the time when my senior high school Chinese literature teacher read in front of the whole class my sample re-constructing writing from a nationwide college entrance examination; in college, my literature professor read my critique to the class as a model example.

For the longest time I did not pay any attention to that. I was driven by this inner drive, led by a dream and desire that I could not even name. I was carried along by the tide of life without much conscious choice of my own, from being a college English teacher at a law school in China to coming to America, pursuing my MBA, and working in corporate America and then in my own business. It was almost like I was sampling life, testing my limits as to how far I could go until the day I was seriously burned out with nothing left to give. In retrospect, that was a message sent by my soul, telling me I had run off course too far and for too long. So it was time for me to get back on track with my life's true meaning. That message was loud, but not so clear to me back then. Loud in the sense that I physically and mentally could not keep living the way I was living, driven by my ego in meeting life's demands.

I often wondered what had happened to me. *Where did my happiness go? What did I do wrong? What is wrong with me? How come I look like a truck ran me over?* The growing awareness that I was my own destiny gave me hope and clarity. It offered me the resolution that enabled me to start the fourth chapter of my life with passion, purpose, and my natural gift of relating to my audience with the universal message of healing. Ever since, I have been passionately inspiring my tribe to be the wholesome people they are by living lives of health in totality.

It is imperative you live the life you are meant to live. Send your subconscious mind a clear signal that you are at peace within, with no conflicting actions that derive from the misalignment of inner and outer. The reason we keep coming back is that we are compelled to neutralize the negative impressions imprinted on our subconscious mind in previous lives. The way to neutralize those negative imprints is to do things that you are born to do, with hints from your deepest desires, wishes, and dreams, which are guided by your gut intuition. Live boldly, live for yourself and your soul's journey, until you have done enough to fulfill your destiny in the physical form so that the impression in your subconscious becomes balanced, or neutralized. Then, and only then, can you continue your soul's journey without the need to come back to human form again, unless you choose to do so to teach others.

This should be reason enough for you to live in alignment with your calling. Otherwise you will be coming back here again and again, with similar sets of circumstances, similar casts of characters, and similar patterns, until the lessons are learned. This is very clear to me now that I have experienced the highs that come from living authentically, though just the happiness and expansiveness spurring through me is reason enough to live life with purpose and meaning. You are here anyway, so you might as well make it count while having fun on this trip called life.

The other huge benefit of living with passion and purpose is that your chance of getting burned out is greatly reduced. Burnout happens when your ego and your true self separate, and your ego takes charge with its own agenda without the true source of energy as backup. When inner and outer are aligned, you operate from that true energy source, tapping into the universal energy and power. You never again have the experience of running on empty, ending up exhausted and fatigued with nothing more to give or offer. When you act from this permanent source of energy, creation, and endless possibility, you are replenished with renewed vigor and vitality, going about your day with the youthful vibrancy that is your birthright.

You start to think, *Maybe there is something here, something I can do with the special gifts and talents I have, and make something out of it. But what is it?* Your antenna is up. Your ears pick up things quickly when people say certain things. You start searching newspaper ads and the internet, looking for something out there that will utilize your passion and gifts. That is what was happening to me when I found the Health Coach Training Program at IIN. I was searching for something that would utilize the organic, wholesome healing I had experienced, my other life experiences and gifts, and my writing and relatedness with people. What could be more rewarding than teaching about what transformed my life and the lives of many others?

Now you are really excited, as I was, suddenly coming alive. Yet fearful thoughts creep in from time to time. *Why do I want to be different from those around me? Is it much easier to just hide behind busyness and numbness? Is it much easier to just zip up and keep all the knowledge to myself? What if I make a fool of myself? Worse yet, what if I change my mind? What if I am wrong?* So you might back off and hide behind your comfortable misery for a while longer. But that deep yearning and unsatisfying feeling keeps you restless. You have to live your purpose; live that life you are born to live; quest for that undying desire. Contentment and satisfaction follow as soon as you make this leap of faith. Excitement and fear follow you around. You know for sure that you are on the right path. You feel the fear and act anyway. You are not in just-surviving mode anymore. You are living, and you are alive! You are thriving! Welcome to the club!

Your life purpose, or the life you are meant to live, comes equipped with the gifts and talents to go with it. Or maybe your passion is so burning hot that it gives you the gumption and desire to learn the skill set needed to make it a reality. Now you are living your dream, where your passion and talent meet, to set you on the road to doing something that is bigger than you, satisfying your deepest desire as well as your sustaining needs, while benefiting the world at large. Now you are on the path to your greatness, with an intensified sense of joy and exhilaration. You are living your purpose.

It is okay to get lost again. It is okay to change your mind. It is okay if you are wrong. It is okay to make a fool of yourself. Living your purpose is not about living a perfect life; rather it is about living the experiences that yield the maximum exhilaration that comes from stretching out of your comfort zone. You are the judge and destiny-maker of your life. If you say it is enough, it is enough. If you feel happiness, you are happy. If you are excited and scared, you are alive. When you stretch out of your comfort zone, you find what you want in your life. Enjoy the stretching, though, because that's part of walking your journey.

Now that you have become your path, check in with yourself constantly. Your guidance is your feeling of contentment and satisfaction, knowing that you are doing what you are supposed to be doing in your life. This is what success is. It is when inner and outer align, with the inner shining through the outer and the outer manifesting the inner as a union.

On days when things are not going as smoothly as you would like, be patient. Stick with the people or things that take your vibration higher. Stay away from the naysayers and downers for the time being, even though they might be here for you to see the part of you that you would rather not see.

When you are aligned with your deepest desires, you are living with your true authenticity. There is no need to be what you are not. Eventually you start to feel like "enough" in your own right. You feel secure without the need to see admiration in others' eyes. You can just be you and attract the forces that are drawn to you. Realizing that I can just be me, and there is no need to prove anything, has been a huge revelation for me. I can simply show up, be free, be light, and be happy.

Once this purpose piece falls into place, it is so much easier to build up your body and energy reserves, since now you are pumped up and have a good reason to be at your most healthy and vibrant. Because of your purpose, meaning, and desire to go on such a journey, this work becomes the journey itself, which shifts seemingly difficult times into ease and grace. Life no longer is a struggle. It becomes effortless grace, infused with a steady, strong, burning fire that is inextinguishable.

There are times when it is essential to do something you may not be so crazy about. But as one fortune cookie says, "To see the rainbow, you have to tolerate the rain." But who says you can't dance in the rain? Everything does not need to be a means to an end. It can be the end by itself when you give it your full presence – body, mind, heart, and soul.

Whatever you are meant to do, you will find the gifts and talents you need to do it, or they will find their way to you in the form of creation or the desire to do that something once you start being aware. Daily, deep connections through various means such as meditation help shed light on what is needed. You have to find this out for yourself. Only you know your truth, and you are unique in your own light, with your set of talents, your purpose, and your own voice and the expression of it.

Here are some things to keep in mind when digging deep into your life's meaning and purpose:

- **Let what you naturally gravitate towards be your guide**. These are the things that get your blood running: things others say that quickly prick up your ears; things that light up your eyes; things that speak to you; things that ignite the fire inside you; things that render you restless and deeply unsatisfied if you don't pursue them; things you would gladly do for free; books you are instantly attached to; topics that draw you in; hobbies you do for leisure; dreams you have at night; answers to questions such as "What would you do if you had all the money and time in the world?" You might say you would go on a vacation and never work another day in your life. But the truth is that you really are not working if you are doing something you enjoy doing. Once your equilibrium returns to normal, you are naturally going to have deeper wants.

- **Journaling and dream recording** are very good ways of discovering your own patterns, hidden gifts, talents, and passions. There are many people teaching just that. "Morning Pages" from Julia Cameron, author of *The Artist's Way,* is a great practice. You simply download everything that runs through your mind first thing in the morning, without filtering. Certain gifts and talents might come to you naturally, while others might need to work at them. Reflect on things you did in school or at work that always got you some recognition. Ask people who know you to tell you about you. If you like to post on social media, your social media friends might tell you a lot about you, too.

- **Love what you do**. Now that you know your gift and passion, find ways to apply them either at work or at your own business, in your own way. Find ways to love what you are currently doing. Sometimes it is just a switch in perspective, like the distribution business I have been talking about. It took the perspective of my friend, seeing it as "free exercise while getting paid to visit friends" for me to see it in a different light. Now I have more reasons to love my distribution business and all it entails. Some of my customers expressed a willingness to sell this book in the most prominent space in their stores. On top of that, they provide me with fertile ground for my constant talking about health, abundance, happiness, choices, awareness, and the here and now.

Always look for a deeper meaning or association with what you are currently doing. For example, one good reason you do what you are currently doing is to sustain you and your family and fund your new passion. It is imperative for you to love what you are currently doing because your health and your happiness depend on it. You might not be able to follow your dreams right away; maybe the switch is going to be a long-term process, maybe your entire life. But if you are not happy with what you are doing, or downright angry every time you perform the tasks, it is going to send signals to your brain transforming that into stress in your body. Our emotions do show up as bodily symptoms, sooner or later, through the intricate body-mind mechanism. That is why it is critical to understand what you are thinking and feeling, and why are you thinking the way you are thinking and feeling the way you are feeling. It is no big surprise that those who have some meaning and purpose in their lives are normally healthier, happier, and live longer, carrying with them the radiance that draws us all in.

My friend Dinah Lin, author of *Daring to Dream Once Again*, comes to mind. Her life is about living her dreams. At seventy-three, she has started the fifth chapter of her life, becoming an author and speaker. She is the embodiment of youth and fire.

- **Do what you love**. Maybe you have exhausted all sources for finding love in what you are currently doing and you still come out with nothing. You simply can't even entertain the idea of doing that again. The very idea of it makes you sick, wanting to throw up. Then the answer is pretty clear: quit and find ways to make your passion work. If you have funds stashed away, then just be with your passion. If you don't have funds available, then obviously you need to look for some solutions for sustaining means.

  I dedicated most of my weekends, holidays, weekday mornings, and weeknights to my passion and life purpose while holding down the distribution business. And the part of my life with the business fell into the big picture of me as a healer, too. You can do what I have been doing: visualize the life you want for yourself, figure out all the pieces that need to come together to make this life a reality, then live in it by taking daily bite-sized actions, making steady and tangible progress. The beauty is you don't need to know all the answers. You simply need to get started.

If your passion is a subject you are familiar with from your life's work or a hobby, find a way to exchange that energy with some income. To me, energy exchange is the basic law of this universe. You give. You receive. Maybe you can teach what you know. Maybe you can write a book about it. Maybe you can sell certain products you are passionate about. Maybe you can teach what you know through a home study course. Maybe you can become a coach. If the subject is new to you, dedicate some time to studying it, either in a structured school or by just reading up on it. In this day and age, all the materials you need are probably at your fingertips for anything you have a fancy for. In tandem, you can come up with a plan or some idea for how to move your passion into a business where you can do it full time and serve more people. This world needs your gift. It is essential to make a good living doing what you love. Otherwise it can be challenging to help those who can benefit from your gift while you are struggling, worrying about your next meal or next month's mortgage.

Start with the act of getting into the knack of it. Gradually transform it into something that can support you and your family while fully stepping into your magnificence and light. If the process is slow, so be it. It is your life, and you don't need to compete with anyone as long as you are being supported by any means applicable to you, and you are living your dream. It sure beats dying a little each day.

Once you have gained clarity and have structures in place, the money will come as a by-product of doing what you love and serving your community, your tribe, and humanity at large. You just need to keep at it, figuring out what works and what does not. That includes marketing as well. You can always leverage your passion by using someone else's structure, either in the form of a job, a partnership, or just a hobby. That really is not as important as fulfilling your deepest desire by living it. You will know. Your heart and your intuition will guide you.

Jack London, the famous writer of the book *The Call of the Wild*, had a passion to be a writer. He taught himself how to read and write while working as a laborer to make a living. He divided his free time into two parts, one part to teach himself how to read, the other part to teach himself how to write by writing a few hours every day before he went to his manual work. Fully use the bits of time others use watching TV, partying, and wasting life away in blindness, while you are soaking up all you can to your heart's content about that thing that makes your blood run faster, your creative juices flow, your heart sing, your face glow, and your whole being alive.

- ***Life purpose* doesn't necessarily mean it is going to be one big thing for the rest of your life**. It can be different from time to time. It could be the smile you automatically flash to that stranger who happens to look your way. It could be the listening ear offered to a friend in need of being heard. It could be the pat on the shoulder for your partner or an encouraging word for a temporary setback.

Life's meaning can be the combination of many small things, which is the case for most people, though we are different in our own ways. It can be different in different phases of your life. It is important to constantly focus on your inner deepest wishes, dreams, and desires. Observe on a regular basis your responses to questions such as "What turns you on?" "What gets your creation going?" "What makes you happy to the point of bliss and exhilaration?" Life lived this way is pure bliss in the making.

Chapter Seven

Sleep Well

Nothing can replace the value of good, old-fashioned, natural sleep. You get up when you naturally wake up, feeling refreshed and energized. It is normally about eight hours, give or take, depending on personal need based on your lifestyle, the degree of stress in your life, how balanced your internal homeostasis is, the amount in your energy-reserve bank account, your biology, etc.

It is definitely more beneficial to come out of sleep naturally, without the startling sound of an alarm o'clock or anything else to drag you out of your peaceful rejuvenation. This gives your body the opportunity to go through the whole cycle of sleeping, from shallow to deep to dream state and into the state of gradually waking up, and reap the benefits. You know firsthand how it feels to have a good night's sleep, getting up feeling recharged, clearheaded, and ready to embrace the day with contentment and smiles. On the other hand, you must have had days when you didn't sleep well. You get up feeling like you were hit by a freight train, more tired than when you went to sleep, fatigued, lifeless, grouchy, and just wishing you could go right back to sleep again, never mind the day and what lies ahead.

When I lack sleep or have poor-quality sleep, you don't want to be around me. I tend to be edgy, easily annoyed, and ready to jump at anyone who appears to be too demanding, uncooperative, or disagreeable. When I do have a good night's sleep, in conjunction with my morning meditation and yoga, push-ups, and a morning cup of *qi* (气功, the cultivation of our life-giving energy), I am bouncy, resilient, happy, and understanding. I am able to put myself in others' shoes, look at things from their perspective, and feel for them. During the day I am full of vitality and presence, and embrace situations that might seem challenging. These, in turn, afford me another good night's sleep. It is a very good cycle with one feeding the other. That is the cycle you want to get into.

Many people look at sleep as wasting chunks of valuable time that can be used to do more important things. But your body depends on the right amount of quality sleep to keep your whole system in balance, your body functioning at its optimal level, and your immunity at its best. I know from experience that all too often we have a tendency to override our bodies' basic needs and jam more things into our already busy lives, attempting to get things done while depleting our sleep quality or time. It is essential to have a good grasp of what sleep can do for you and to give it top priority, not compromising sleep time for anything. Here are some of the benefits of quality sleep:

- **Deep, restful sleep resets your system, the way your computer is reset by turning it off and then back on, so that you can start a new day refreshed.** Sleeping is essential for maintaining and resetting your equilibrium – the natural balanced state your body needs to function properly. Thus it can work as the well-functioning, coherent system it is, assisting you in carrying out your daily tasks to create and live the life you dream of living. Your body's equilibrium helps it perform its innate, involuntary functions of keeping itself alive, such as absorbing nourishment, making good quality blood, growing new cells, pumping blood, maintaining the beautiful rhythm of your heartbeat, keeping your body temperature at its most ideal, and transporting oxygen to all parts of your body through the flow of blood and vital, life-energy *qi*.

- **Quality sleep helps restore and repair some of the oxidized or damaged cells that result from performing normal functions such as breathing, moving, eating, thinking, feeling, acting, and the other activities of our stress-loaded, hectic modern living.** Scientists understand that both phases of sleep, REM – rapid eye movement and NREM – the deep sleep afterward, are essential in revitalizing and restoring mental functions as well as physiological bodily functions. While REM sleep energizes your brain, the deep phases of sleep following REM provide a more rejuvenating state of rest where your blood pressure drops, you breathe more deeply and slowly, your brain rests deeply, and more blood is directed to the muscles and cells in the body, assisting in repairing, restoring, and growing.

- **Quality sleep also helps rejuvenate muscles and generate new cells.** Your pituitary gland secrets streams of growth hormone, which promote muscle repair and new cell growth once your body gets into the deep, peaceful phases of sleep. Poor quality and shorter duration sleep hinder the release of growth hormone, therefore muscle repair and new cell growth.

- **A proper bedtime schedule fine-tunes, resets, cleanses, renews, and rejuvenates.** Chinese medicine associates internal bodily organs with specific time periods during which they primarily perform certain functions. If you work a traditional daytime schedule, the time after sundown to 1:00am is the best time for your body to make and store blood. So the earlier you go to bed after darkness falls, the more quality blood reserves your body can build up. It is taught by some that if you always go to sleep at 11:00pm, your body will make enough blood to offset what has been consumed, keeping the level at balance with no excess for reserves. This also depends on feeding your body with quality, nourishing meals at the right times and in the right amounts, and on other lifestyle and mindset choices. If you can consistently go to sleep around 9:00pm, your body not only makes enough blood to supply what is being consumed, but is also able to stash some excess into the reserve bank and use some for deeper repairing of earlier damage from stress and unmindful living. This can make up for those occasional days when going to bed at 9:00pm is simply out of the question. Life does happen. Do what you can to build up your blood reserves and the quality of your blood. Your everyday life and your future well-being depend on it. Eleven pm through 1:00am is associated with gall bladder health. It is the beginning stage in the cleansing of tissues, processing cholesterol, and setting the stage for the liver time – 1:00am to 3:00am – for the cleansing of blood and the processing of waste. The lung hours – 3:00am to 5:00am – are when respiration, oxygenation, and expulsion of waste gasses take place. This is a time when the blood takes the *qi*-intake of oxygen to all parts of the body, bringing with it the vital energy for the day's functioning. It is also a time to get rid of waste gasses and connect with the higher spirit with each breath.

- **Sleeping connects you with your spiritual realm through dreams.** We all have dreams so vivid, so real, and so emotional we literally can feel them. Some dreams are simply not of this world. This is your soul's way of telling you something about the journey you are on – the emotions, past lives, and unresolved tangles that require your attention. That is why so many people write dream journals, jotting dreams down right after getting up while the memory still lingers. This can be life-changing. It can assist you in unlocking what has been holding you back, unleashing more potential, and making this life count. The other benefit of connecting with source during deep sleep is that you get replenished by the source with all its rejuvenating qualities, which we covered extensively in the chapter about meditation.

In short, the benefits are many. It is as important as good, nutritious, and delicious food, the movement of your body, the way you think and feel, your general outlook towards life, and your way of being.

One of my acquaintances felt sick and didn't want to eat. All the medical tests and doctor's visits could not solve anything. But after a good night's sound sleep, all the symptoms were gone. He was as good as new.

We have all seen people burn the late-night oil, watching TV, partying, or just catching up on piled-up work without much consideration for the detrimental effect it has on their health. From a cell's perspective, lost sleep can never be made up. What's lost is lost forever. Insufficient sleep shows up in the body as aging, stress, tiredness, impaired immunity function, and the stubborn excess weight that won't go away. Establish a reasonable sleep schedule and stick to it as much as possible. Then you at least have something to borrow from on days when you are depleting your reserves. Here are some suggestions to keep you well restored, energized, and refreshed through a good night's rejuvenating sleep:

- **Stay busy during the day to ensure a good night's sleep.** Life, in a sense, is very fair in that things have to balance out. If you use the full capacity of your body, your brain, or a combination of both, you are rewarded with a good night's sound sleep. So be happy you are alive and vibrant, able to work your muscles during the day, and then sink deeply into a night of rejuvenating sleep with a sense of satisfaction, coziness, and contentment.

- **Don't do anything right before bedtime that will get you excited so that you can't fall asleep.** I choose not to do anything creative right before bedtime, such as serious writing, working on marketing, or anything stimulating that will get me going. If I do, my brain gets so fired up that it won't calm down until late into the night, which costs me the best time for falling asleep, not to mention the damage it does to my body and my wellness the next day. For some people it is sports of any sort that gets them going. Find out what it is for you, and make sure you don't do it. Do something that brings on sleepiness and gets you ready for a good night's sleep, such as light reading. I can't start reading a good novel and stop in the middle, so I stick with non-fiction reading.

- **Do some yoga, qigong, or meditation.** They all help you get to the natural state of wakeful awareness, preparing you for deeper sleep. I often find myself drifting into unconsciousness while deep in meditation, which is my body's way of telling me that I am ready for deep sleep. I just take the cue from my body and don't fight it, extending my rest from restful awareness into restful sleep. I usually change my position from sitting to lying down, which allows my body to send the signal that I am at complete rest and that no fight-or-flight hormone is needed for the time being. I often don't use a pillow; I just lay my head on the mattress, which positions my head at the same level as my body, giving it a good chance to fully rest.

- **Don't ingest anything other than a light drink for three to four hours, or at least two hours, before your usual bedtime.** Food needs blood for digestion, and eating late interferes with your blood's usual nighttime task of cleansing, making more blood, resetting, repairing, restoring, regenerating, and building. Not only will the food affect your quality of sleep, but it will also lead to weight gain resulting from sluggish digestion. Be very mindful of drinking as well. If you are waking up because of nature's call to empty your bladder, it is better not to drink before bedtime. Drink water long before bedtime, giving it the chance to run through your system before you fall asleep.

- **Keep your room properly aired and slightly cool by turning down the heat a couple of degrees.** It will help your body's built-in mechanism for cooling down your core body temperature to effectively sleep, ensuring a night of restfulness, peacefulness, and complete rejuvenation.

- **Make a habit of keeping your bedtime schedule from around 9:00pm to 5:00am (if you work a traditional daytime schedule).** Eastern wellness philosophies reinforce the importance of living in harmony with nature, rising with the sunrise, and resting with the sunset. That is how I was brought up as a child growing up in the countryside in China at a time when there was no electricity. The saying "Early to bed and early to rise makes a man healthy, wealthy, and wise" applies. So does the Chinese saying "Early to rise, early to bed creates good health." The quality of your sleep will be so much better, so much more restorative than a 12:00 midnight to 8:00 in the morning routine. Even though they are both eight hours, the former offers more rejuvenation benefit, while the latter actually weakens your bodily functions since it is in disharmony with nature and the sunrise-sunset cycle.

Once you understand what poor sleep is doing to your body, you will work out a way to keep a reasonable bedtime schedule. Once it becomes a habit, it will be effortless. I look forward to my rejuvenating sleep after some connecting in the stillness of wakeful awareness. If for some reason you wake up at around 4:00 in the morning and you feel you have had enough sleep, don't go back to sleep; you might oversleep, which will cause an adverse effect. When you get up too late in the morning, against nature's rhythm, you can feel sluggish all day. Even if you go to bed late, get up at 5:00am or 6:00am anyway. Stay active during the day, nap a little – about ten to thirty minutes or so right after lunchtime – to carry you through the day. As a matter of fact, I remember taking naps daily when I was in college in China. The practice is still prevalent there, where most people lie down after lunch, have a bit of a nap, and then go about the day again with renewed energy.

- **If you wake up in the middle of the night and can't get back to sleep, simply sit up, close your eyes, travel inside, and let that forever stillness fountain of youth rejuvenate you.** It is the second-best option under the circumstances. Many agree that good rest is comprised of two parts: restful sleep and restful awareness. I find it quite helpful to relax into stillness and immerse in the ever-presence of eternity, allowing myself to be carried over naturally into a night's restful sleep.

Chapter Eight

Feed the Body That Houses Your Soul

1. Hydrate Your Body

Your body is mostly water – over 70 percent. Water is your body's principal element. It makes up about 60 percent of your body weight and is vital for many functions in your body such as flushing toxins out of every organ, carrying nutrients to every part of your body through the bloodstream, keeping your throat and joints moist, and so on. There is a story about a doctor who was shut up in a prison camp along with many other prisoners. One of the prisoners got very sick, and the good doctor could not do anything other than give the patient water. To his surprise, the patient got better. He cured many prisoners with similar conditions in the same way. After he got out of prison, he focused on using water as a cure.

Dr. F. Batmanghelidj is that doctor. He wrote about his "water cure." At Watercure.com he says:

> You're not sick; you're thirsty. Don't treat thirst with medication…Water is the basis of all life and that includes your body. Your muscles that move your body are 75% water; your blood that transports nutrients is 82% water; your lungs that provide your oxygen are 90% water; your brain that is the control center of your body is 76% water; even your bones are 25% water.

The water in your body is consumed or lost throughout the day through the skin, breathing, sweat, urination, and excretion, and the lost water needs to be replenished. On hot days, more water in the body evaporates through sweat than on cool days, especially if you are moving around quite a bit outdoors. In winter, water is pulled out of your body to balance dry conditions around you. The heating system in your house and at work further dries out your respiratory system. You are what you drink. Water is your lifeline. Be sure to replenish the water in your body throughout the day.

- **Sip hot water throughout the day**. To stay hydrated, develop the habit of sipping water throughout the day, beginning as soon as you get up in the morning. The Eastern tradition emphasizes sipping hot water, in that hot water matches up with the internal digestive fire; therefore it fans the fire to burn stronger, yielding better digestion. Hot water penetrates deep into the pores, hydrating the body thoroughly, while cold water runs through the body quickly without being taken up by the deep cells in the body. Many believe the best remedy for constipation is sipping plain-old hot water throughout the day with nothing added to it. Boiled water is purely H_2O, with nothing else left, the state of water that deep cells accept for hydration.

Many say older people die not of old age, but of dehydration and hunger due to the body's inability to extract water and nutrients from food and liquids. After I started reversing my body's symptoms of illness, I picked up the habit of sipping hot water right after my morning meditation to start my day. It is usually plain boiled water, or with fresh lemon and pure honey on days when my throat feels dry, chrysanthemum tea on days when I feel an internal flare building up, fresh ginger tea on days when I feel up to building up my yang energy, or sometimes another non-caffeinated hot drink.

- **Don't wait until you are thirsty to drink.** By then the imbalance has developed. Keep sipping water throughout the day.

- **Keep a large bottle of water with you, ideally the stainless steel type.** There are times when you may not be able to avoid using bottled water, but limit your exposure whenever you can. There is evidence that plastic bottles, under extreme cold and hot conditions, leech cancer-causing chemicals into the water. There are many ways the water can get exposed to extreme temperatures between the bottling plant and the store. I have seen bottled water for sale sitting in a window in the heat or outside the store exposed to direct sun in the peak of summer. I was told once that the claim about carcinogens leeching from plastic is a political one, but even if bottled water is safe to consume, the fact that the plastic bottles are not biodegradable is reason enough to avoid them.

- **Water content in soups, vegetables, fruits, and other foods counts as water intake.** Ingestion of vegetables, watermelons, and many other fruits rich in water content is beneficial. Be mindful of fruits, though, as they are high in sugar content.

- **In America, water from the faucet is safe enough as drinking water, even though many disagree.** You can always invest in a water filtration system. It's important to understand what you are getting. I have given up drinking anything other than boiled water, hot or room temperature. If there should be any bacteria remaining after all the treatment before the water gets to your pipes, boiling will for sure take care of that. Buy a nice-looking water kettle. Then all your water needs will be taken care of. In the summer keep some boiled, cooled water either in the kettle or in a glass jar for daily use. You can even refrigerate it if you really love the coldness, as so many people do. Just sip, instead of drinking it fast, which gives your body a chance to warm it up before the water reaches your digestive tract, so as not to impact your digestive fire as much. You can always add lemon, or chrysanthemum, or even raw ginger (if it is before noon) when the water is boiling hot, then you'll have the natural and healthy flavored drink you like once cooled down. A word of caution about ginger: According to Chinese wellness philosophy, ginger ingested in the morning works as ginseng in the body, building and nourishing, whereas it acts as a poison in the body when taken at night. So be sure to drink ginger tea only in the early part of the day.

- **Caffeinated drinks such as tea and coffee actually deplete your body of its water content, causing your body to lose more water than it actually takes in by pulling water out of your cells.** If you feel you need a cup of coffee or tea in the morning to give you a boost, you have some serious digging and adjusting to do in your lifestyle, your food choices, and the way you assimilate your emotions and thoughts. Caffeine robs your body of energy reserves you may or may not have. Drinking coffee or tea first thing in the morning is sort of like borrowing money from the already depleted energy bank account. Here you are stimulating your body to make more energy from a negative energy balance. This is where energy consumption is more than the energy being built up. Your health is in the declining stage. Your body is in no position to provide the energy boost. Consistent long-term depletion leads to severe fatigue and weight gain, and can even lead to depression. Coffee and tea do have their good antioxidant properties; just don't drink them first thing in the morning without food. A better idea is to have coffee with your lunch. You will also benefit from its stimulating factor to better digest your food while you savor its rich aroma.

- **Avoid sugary drinks, including soda and juice.** I once watched a short video of a young man walking around Manhattan to burn off the calories ingested from a sixteen-ounce soft drink. At first he was energetic, happy, and walking fast. His steps gradually started to slow down, even dragged. Towards the end he had a hard time putting one foot in front of the other. Many people have had the experience of running on a treadmill, watching the slow burn-up of calories. It takes quite some effort to burn off even a few calories. So never entertain the idea that you are active, you move a lot, and therefore you can have that sugary stuff. These drinks have loads of empty calories, meaning calories with no nutritional value to back them up. In other words, you are filling your body up and getting yourself sick without the benefit of any useful fuel for your body, your cells, and your muscles to draw on. These drinks trigger binge eating too, since your body seeks real, sustaining nutrients even though your belly might be full.

  Next time you want to drink a can of soda, slow down and read the calorie content. I am not a big fan of counting calories in everyday living; I am just emphasizing this to demonstrate a point. If you are going to go for something that is sugary, go for naturally sweet foods. At least they give your body something it needs while you indulge. It is important that you understand this. I knew some people who lost quite a lot of weight in the waistline because they had stopped drinking soda. I also met people who complained to me that they didn't seem able to get rid of the excessive weight given the fact that they ate very little; they drank sugary, caffeinated drinks. The combination of eating very little and drinking soft drinks is the easiest way to gain weight, simply because all the excess empty calories are stored as body fat. Meanwhile your cells are constantly looking for good fuels to give you the energy to function on a daily basis. Without that energy, and with an empty energy reserve bank, your body simply does not have the strength to burn off these empty calories, leaving you heavy and unhappy.

- **Many factors play a role in the right quantity of water to drink.** It varies with your body build, your health, your activity level, and even the season of the year. You might have heard the advice of drinking 8 glasses (about 1.9 liters) of fluids per day, which is more or less in line with the recommendation from the Institute of Medicine to drink about 13 cups (3 liters) of total beverage a day for men and 9 cups (2.2 liters) of total beverage a day for women. Obviously, when you are outside in the summer gardening or cutting grass, you certainly want to drink more to replenish the water lost through sweat. You probably feel like drinking more water in a heated house during the winter with the heat drying you out. As long as you feel hydrated, and your urine looks clear or light yellow, you are fine. When you feel a swelling in your

> stomach, then you know you have more than enough water. The common sense approach is the best. Listen to your body. Let it be your guide, as it should be for everything else in life.

A properly hydrated body stays younger longer with more vigor, youthfulness, and younger-looking skin. Don't forget that water today.

2. Nourish Your Body with Good, Wholesome Foods

When I was growing up, I remember a time when life was getting better, and people started to have whiter and whiter steamed bread. In the process of separating the bran and germ (the outer layer and the reproductive part of the wheat kernel that germinates and forms the wheat grass, both of which contain fibers and oil) from the endosperm (the inner ball of starch), more of the rough part was being separated from the white starchy part. The process takes longer with a horse walking circles around a giant stone mill. Normally there were only two piles in the end, one dark and one fine. The dark pile was the rough part of the skin and the germ used to feed the family animals, mostly pigs, while the finer part was mostly from the endosperm and was for the family. At some point people began to mill three separate piles: one rough one for the pigs, a medium one for the family, and the finest part was reserved for the very old and very young or for guests and special occasions.

Back then, the whiter the flour, the better quality it was perceived to be. The whiter your family bread or your noodles, the more prestige they held or the richer you were. Neighbors would say you had it made when your bread was whiter. My mother started complaining of indigestion and her stomach bloating. She constantly commented, "We poor people do not have much good fortune in life. We cannot even digest the whiter bread made out of the more refined flour." The stools even smelled foul and became finer, thinner, and less in volume. For the longest time I never gave it much thought. During my study at IIN, it finally occurred to me what had been happening.

Whole foods provide our body all it needs: protein, carbohydrates, fats, minerals, and vitamins. Digesting food starts with the chewing of food in the mouth, then it goes through the esophagus down to the stomach and to the small intestine – the major site for nutrient absorption; the remainder then moves to the large intestine where the microbiomes living in your gut wall feed on some fibers and the rest is removed through the excretion of stool. In the process, the nutrients in the food have been absorbed into the bloodstream as building blocks and are carried to all parts of the body, sustaining, supporting, building, and repairing.

In ideal conditions, we eat food in its natural form with some degree of processing, such as cooking, to aid in digestion. Our body takes all it needs – some for storage, the rest goes out of the body as waste, sweeping up along the way some dead cells; used, dirty cholesterol; undigested matter; dead bacteria; and toxins, leaving the body clean and functioning at peak level. Fibers naturally come with whole foods. There are soluble fibers and insoluble fibers. Soluble fibers such as the ones occurring in oats and most fruits absorb water while insoluble fibers occurring mostly in grains and vegetables remain intact. The soluble fibers soak up water, help build up stools from undigested matter, and scoop up dead cells, dead bacteria, and used cholesterol along the digestive tract, while the insoluble fibers push through, normally within twenty-four hours. When the fibers, both soluble and insoluble, have been stripped off the foods before eating, stool becomes thinner and less frequent, resulting in poor toxin removal. The buildup of toxicity in the body shows up as deposits in fat tissues and facial skin, leading to the onset of many modern-day diseases.

Every disease can be traced back to poor digestion, therefore lifestyle and food choices. When food is refined, where oil, fiber, and protein are removed and only the starchy content is left (such as in the case of white rice and refined flour), your body's functioning becomes sluggish. Digestion is less than ideal, causing bloating and other digestive disorders. The chain of digestive malfunction needs to be broken, starting with wholesome, mindful food choices.

This whole business of eating healthy can be summed up in one sentence: Eat wholesome mostly plant-based real foods in moderation. As Michael Pollen puts it in *In Defense of Food: An Eater's Manifesto*: "Eat food. Not too much. Mostly plants."

(a) Add More Vegetables

Vegetables are a very nutritious choice to include in your diet – vegetables of various shapes and all the colors of the rainbow carry the phytonutrients (nutrients from plants) that are derived from the sun's life energy. Use varieties that add color, texture, aroma, nutrition, and diversity to your meals. Eat more vegetables that are in season.

There is a theory originating from *food energetics* that says that the organs benefit most from vegetables with a shape similar to that of the organ. Heart-shaped vegetables are good for the heart. Leafy greens with all their veins benefit the respiratory system and improve circulation. Experiment with this theory. As long as you use moderation as your guideline, your intuition as your guide, and learn about your *bio-individuality* (more about this in chapter eight) and specific vegetables over time, you should do just fine.

Leafy greens are really good choices in that they are low in calories; full of vitamins and minerals; good for building, cleansing, and digestion; promote circulation; and help alleviate constipation. Good digestion is the foundation for good nutrients to be assimilated and absorbed by the body. It helps the respiratory system with all its veins, sending oxygen to all parts of the body. If you normally don't have leafy greens in your diet, start experimenting with some. It is always good to start somewhere. If you regularly eat leafy greens, expand the varieties and quantities. You can eat as much as you would like without concern about any detrimental effects. This is the one "free" food you can enjoy, as greens are calorie-light and nutrient-dense, meaning they offer loads of nutritional value without many calories. Leafy greens in spring, freshly sprung out of the ground, are the best natural remedy for cleansing and assisting in removing accumulated toxins out of your body from a whole winter's intake of relatively heavy food keeping you insulated from the bitter cold.

Dandelion is a really good spring detoxifier. Rich in potassium, iron, magnesium, and various vitamins, it is also a diuretic, enhancing the activities of the kidney and liver. It pulls water out in the form of increased urination from areas where there is excess water building up causing swelling or edema. It can assist in naturally addressing water retention in any part of the body, in the meanwhile flushing out unwanted toxins. It is considered a natural remedy for urinary tract infections and has been used in Chinese medicine for thousands of years. I remember picking dandelion from the fields, either to sell to the local collection center or for my mom to make my favorite childhood food, dandelion chunks. These are so mouthwateringly delicious, with a hint of earthy, sweet, and bitter tastes. It is medicine as food and food as medicine in its most beautiful and natural embodiment.

You can also use dandelion in your salads. It is bitter raw, but perfectly safe, as the bitterness is the cleansing agent. You can also bake the roots and leaves and make tea out of them. Have them early in the day, though, to avoid interrupting your sleep with bathroom visits or urinating in bed. If you are not using weed killers, any sort of commercial fertilizers, or any bug killers (pesticides) in your yard, you can do what I just did the other day: pick dandelions from your own backyard instead of buying them at the store. These are actually the best – truly organic in all senses, supported by the local elements, and very beneficial to your body. If you are not sure what they are or you simply don't recognize them, buy them at your local market. You will be surprised what you can find at the market these days.

Low-starch vegetables are in abundant supply. Vegetables like the ones you often see in your local food market: broccoli, zucchini, green beans, cauliflower, celery, etc. While they do have some carbohydrate (starch) content, they also offer good fiber content and are loaded with nutrients. They serve as good fillers in your meals to fill you up and aid in digestion by promoting good stool movement as well as feeding the bugs in your digestive tract. If you eat them first, you will need only very small portions of meat and starch, especially refined starches, until your hormonal signals tell you, "I am full now."

The allium family of vegetables and herbs includes onions of all colors, garlic, scallions, shallots, leeks, and chives. They are known in folklore as ingredients that flavor and have medicinal value. You can find them anywhere and they are very inexpensive. You can buy a five-pound bag of onions for a few dollars and it will last for quite a while. They are loaded with health-promoting and curative benefits, low in calories, and rich in soluble dietary fiber. Due to their anti-inflammatory, antioxidant properties derived from sulfite compounds and quercetin, these vegetables can help lower blood sugar levels in diabetics, decrease blood vessel stiffness, and reduce total blood pressure and overall risk of coronary heart disease. They are also antibacterial, antiviral, anti-carcinogenic, and rich in vitamin C, B-complex, and the mineral manganese. Use them generously in your everyday cooking.

Nightshade vegetables are vegetables that grow mostly during the night, which is how the category gets its name. The ones I know of include eggplant, peppers of various colors, cucumbers, and tomatoes. According to Chinese thinking, nightshade vegetables are yin (female/feminine) by nature, or cooling. Yin is associated with darkness, water, cooling, and nourishment. In a sense these vegetables have the qualities of diuretics. They induce an increase in urination and draw water out of excessively built-up areas. On the other hand, the yin nature can worsen the internal condition of *yin dominance,* where yang is needed for balance. If you urinate very frequently, you might want to avoid eating these vegetables until your condition improves. As long as overall consumption is well balanced, where many different varieties of vegetables and other food combinations are well mixed into your diet, there should be no negative consequence. Keep in mind that the cooking method used alters food energetics. Yin vegetables combined with raw or uncooked foods yield more cooling, while the heat from cooking can neutralize their yin and cooling effect.

Root vegetables are rich in flavonoid antioxidants, vitamins, minerals, and dietary fiber. They are grounding and sustaining by nature. These vegetables are deeply rooted underground, firmly entrenched in the soil, getting their sunshine through the parts of the plant that are above the ground. They are associated with the digestive system, serving as the foundation of health and well-being. Root vegetables include sweet potatoes, carrots, rutabagas, beets, turnips, radishes, and onions. They are starchier than the other vegetables, and sweet potatoes contain the most starch.

> **Potatoes** have been a staple food all over the world, in every culture, throughout history since their distribution from the new world began. They are starchy, loaded with vitamins and minerals, very inexpensive, and can be cooked so many ways! Be it baked, boiled, steamed, sautéed, mashed, diced, or sliced. I always loved my mom's sliced or shredded potatoes sautéed in garlic with vinegar. On WeChat – a Chinese-based social media – I read about various Chinese doctors saying potatoes cooked that way help reduce weight.

Somehow this innocent food has been associated with the rising epidemic of obesity and diabetes. Potatoes are categorized as a vegetable in the USDA Food Pyramid. They are an American favorite, showing up everywhere – in homes, restaurants, supermarkets, even vending machines. But French fries and potato chips ruin it for potatoes. They have trashed potatoes in several ways, especially the white ones. They are deep-fried in corn oil or vegetable oil (soybean oil), which is probably from genetically modified corn or soybeans, or maybe even a small portion (less than 5 percent) of partially hydrogenated oil (trans fat) that has been reused many times over. Potato chips are tortured further with preservatives, artificial flavorings, sugars of all kinds, and who knows what else. They are loaded with calories without anything good for the body, exposing eaters to potential weight gain, sluggish digestion, cancer-causing compounds, aging skin, and fatigue, especially when combined with a sedentary lifestyle and other poor food choices.

Potatoes, like any other wholesome food, are good and wholesome by themselves. Moderation, the overall composition of a meal, and other lifestyle factors all play a role in the rate of absorption into the bloodstream as sugar. Keep the portion moderate, such as a small to medium-sized potato in a meal a few times a week served as a starch. Keep in mind that the white potato was on the 2014 Environmental Working Group's Dirty Dozen list, having the most chemical residue. It makes sense to choose organic over traditional or be sure to cook them well to remove some of the toxins.

Among potatoes, the **red potato** is slower in absorption and relatively cleaner. You may want to use more red potatoes in your home cooking than white. You can oven-bake potatoes, sliced or diced. Put cut pieces on a baking sheet, sprinkle with oil (light olive oil, organic, or 100 percent expeller-pressed corn oil, peanut oil, sunflower oil, or safflower oil – oils with higher smoke points) and a bit of sea salt, and bake in the oven at 350°F for about twenty minutes or until golden brown. I once saw a recipe for potatoes cut into thin slices from the top, not all the way through, still held together at the bottom; drizzle oil, sprinkle the top with salt and black pepper, and bake in the oven at 420° for about forty minutes. They sure beat fried potato chips.

Sweet potatoes are at the top of the list for slower absorption, which makes them the best in the potato family. I have always loved sweet potatoes, even as a child. On many cold winter days, when I came home from school my mother would hand me a roasted sweet potato from the firepit the family used for cooking food. It was so delicious, sweet, toasty, and hearty. I am so glad that they are slower in turning into blood sugar as well.

The potato family is one of nature's good foods. As long as we view them as a good carbohydrate and consume them in moderate amounts in their original form, they are building, satisfying, and sustaining, sticking to the ribs and keeping us fuller longer.

(b) Eat More Unaltered Grains

Whole grains have been staple foods for humans since early civilization. Experiment with incorporating whole grains into meals of any cuisine you are familiar or comfortable with. There is a wide variety of grains available in the United States, with an abundance of supplies from all over the world, such as black rice, brown rice, millet, buckwheat, quinoa, amaranth, and corn. They are all rich in minerals and full of protein, fat, and starch – a whole food all wrapped together in tiny grains. They are very filling. They slow absorption of nutrients into the bloodstream due to the fiber content and assist in keeping sugar level steady, therefore keep you full longer. The fiber from the outer layer not only assists in the timely removal of stool, but feeds the one pound or so of microflora or healthy bacteria residing in your gut wall, aiding in digestion, promoting smooth functioning, and building up immunity.

(c) Incorporate Beans and Legumes

Beans of all varieties, sizes, and colors such as black, white, red, and green (mung beans) are very rich in protein, B vitamins, iron, and fiber. Beans benefit everyone, especially if you are a vegetarian or semi-vegetarian. Watch out for the genetically modified version of soybeans. Discard any broken beans before preparing them. You can cook beans in many different ways based on your preferences and ethnicity. In this big melting pot of culture in America, you can pretty much cook them any way you prefer and make them uniquely yours. Beans need to be thoroughly cooked; *al dente* – cooked to be firm – doesn't work well with beans. They need to be presoaked, brought to a boil, then slow-cooked or simmered for a couple of hours until done. Once they are done, you can use them in salads, soups, wraps, or simply serve them with your meals as starch or protein.

(d) Enjoy Good Fat

Over the years, *fat* has been considered a dirty word. It is associated with obesity and heart disease. That viewpoint is reflected in the USDA food guidelines. In its place are sugar and refined carbohydrates. You have seen all the low-fat versions of packaged foods out there. But somehow 50 percent of Americans are overweight. What has happened?

The truth is, we need fat in our meals to make them taste better and be more satisfying and more sustaining. Of the food groups, fat is the last to be absorbed, therefore keeping us fuller longer. Consumed in conjunction with other food groups, it eases up the absorption of the food into the bloodstream, therefore helping to keep blood sugar level steady. Fat consumption gives the body more energy in the form of backup fuel after the main fuel, carbohydrate, has been burned off. Adequate intake of fat also aids absorption of the fat-soluble vitamins A, D, E, and K, which promote eyesight, strengthen bones by boosting calcium absorption, and protect cells by neutralizing free radicals. Fat cells stored in adipose tissue help insulate your body and keep your core body temperature steady. The key is the right kind of fats:

Clean Meat (more of protein than of fat)

With the spread of factory farms, most livestock is raised commercially, on a large scale, aiming for productivity and the bottom line. Growth hormones are used to facilitate the growth of the animals, shortening the period of feeding at the stockyard. These animals exist in a feedlot that is overly crowded and are injected with antibiotics and vaccines to keep disease to a minimum. To boot, they are fed all sorts of industrialized end-products and corn or soybeans that are heavily sprayed with pesticides with industrial-strength sprayers. Most of these soybean and corn seeds have been genetically modified from the original, natural form, the long-term detrimental effects of which are not known but have been associated with impaired immunity and infertility.

In his book *Deception,* Jeffrey Smith talks about animals bypassing genetically modified feeds and naturally gravitating to traditional non-genetically-modified food sources. Genetically modified foods are associated with the malformation and even death of the animals consuming them. The switch from genetically modified to non-genetically-modified foods reverses the condition. If you eat meat, it pays to eat clean, because you take on the sum and totality of the animals you eat – their life, the food they ingested, and their environment – that has been stored in their cell memory.

When you shop, look for grass-fed meat and organic, pasture-raised, free-range chicken and eggs. At the very least, look for free-range chicken and free-range eggs.

Free-range only means that the animals are not caged. Even if they are outdoors, they might be limited to some areas of dirt. They might be roaming outdoors in green pastures feasting on bugs, but it is not guaranteed unless specifically specified as **pasture-raised** or if you see it yourself when you shop locally. **Organic-raised** only means they are fed organic feed. They could be confined to tight quarters, where the beaks of the chicken are removed, or the tails of the pigs are cut off to prevent them attacking others or being attacked due to the overly tight quarters. Free-range, pasture-raised animals can still be fed with genetically modified corn, soybeans, or any of the industrially treated feeds loaded with chemicals, pesticides, and antibiotics. But they are one step better than animals raised in cramped conditions.

Milk and dairy products are best from organic, grass-fed, free-roaming animals. It is always better to choose whole milk. If you want to ingest less fat, dilute it with water. As for whether to choose raw or pasteurized, I leave it to you. If you have a source for raw milk, you can always boil it at home before drinking. It is actually quite delicious that way, warming and cozy.

Seafood is best wild-caught and quick-frozen if you do not have the convenience and luxury of living close to a clean waterway with no industrial dumping or serious pollution. Farm-raised seafood has some of the same problems as farm-raised livestock – close-quartered and being fed conventional feed. Choose smaller fish as well, since the toxic buildup in them is not as heavy. Large tuna are loaded with mercury, and prolonged and frequent consumption can lead to a toxic level of mercury in your body. Pinkish-orange salmon is said to contain fewer toxins.

Know your source and your food by exploring local animal farms where animal meat is sold. Go visit them to see how they treat their animals. What do they feed them? Are the animals healthy and happy? It is always good to know the source of the feed as well. The best is grass-fed, with some additional organic or non-genetically-modified feed.

You can certainly raise your own meat if you are able, willing, and have space. I remember when I was growing up we had pigs, chickens, horses, cows, and sheep in the yard. It was commonly part of the domestic scene – a way of life. If you do this you can have fresh milk, eggs, chicken, or red meat and share, barter, or sell the balance to your neighbors. It can even become a lifestyle.

Good Oils

Oils add flavor, satiety, and fullness to meals while providing heart and brain benefits. Be sure to use good oils and stay away from the unhealthy ones. Always keep your oil tightly covered and stored in a dark, cool place, avoiding oxidation.

Olive oil has more oleic acid or more monounsaturated (omega-9) fatty acids and polyphenols, rendering it more resistant to oxidation. It is heart-healthy and can assist in lowering blood pressure and cholesterol. There are several varieties of olive oil derived from either cold pressing or filtering and refining. Extra virgin olive oil is the purest, from the first pressing; virgin olive oil is from the second pressing; and pure olive oil is a combination of pressed and refined. There are other mixes of oils labeled as olive oil. Always be sure to read the ingredients and extraction method. It is one of the healthiest of oils, and is more expensive than most others. It has a relatively low burning point, so high-temperature cooking leads to deterioration and a pronounced bitter taste. It is best cooked at a low temperature, as in sautéing, or used on salads or in cold dishes. Refined olive oil is perfectly suited for high-temperature cooking such as frying or baking.

Coconut oil: I have been using coconut oil for almost all of my heated cooking, including sautéing. It is satisfying, gratifying, delicious, heart- and brain-healthy, and benefits eaters with a natural food loaded with about 90 percent saturated fat from medium-chain fatty acids. It goes directly to the liver from the digestive tract as quick energy or is turned into ketone bodies (water-soluble molecules produced by the liver from fatty acids at times of low food or low carbohydrate intake for cells of the body to use as energy), delivering therapeutic effects on brain disorders. It is one of the few *superfoods*.

Nut and seed oils are now seen more often on the shelves of food stores. They are very beneficial as well, sharing the benefits of their seed origins. Peanut oil and almond oil can be used for heated cooking. Sesame, walnut, and flaxseed oil are best used in low-temperature or cold dishes such as salads. Flaxseed oil is easily oxidized, so instead of buying the oil, purchase flaxseeds, store them in a cool place, and grind them down on a per-use basis. Read the label on the seed package for more instructions.

Canola oil is rich in omega-3 fatty acids, with a ratio of 2 to 1 of omega-6 to omega-3. It is made from rapeseed by a refining process using hexane after the seeds have been slightly heated and crushed. Some say the name comes from Can(ada)ola(oil), while others say it is Can(ada)+o(il)+l(ow)+a(cid). Oil from traditionally grown crops seems to be safe and healthy, despite what I have heard about the issues of rapeseed, hexane, and erucic acid. The main issue seems to be that the oil is derived from genetically modified crops. Suggestions seem to point to using **organic, expeller-pressed canola oil**, which eliminates the concern about erucic acid, hexane, and genetic modification; it might be more expensive because the expeller press extracting method is less efficient than using hexane solvent. The majority of crops are genetically modified, about 87 percent in the US and about 90 percent in Canada. ***But if you can find the organic version, it is cheaper than olive oil and coconut oil and offers a higher smoke point of 425°F, ideal for high-temperature cooking.***

Refined soybean and corn oil are very inexpensive, offering a higher smoke point of 450°, ideal for frying and baking needs. ***Be sure to choose oils from organic crops***. Avoid buying oils from genetically modified crops. Chances are good that canola, soybean, and corn oil from your grocery store are from genetically modified crops if not specifically labeled as organic. Pay close attention to the labeling.

(e) Spice Up Your Meals

Spices not only have good nutritional properties, they are also medicinal. On top of adding flavor to your foods, spices make them more appealing, more enticing, more appetizing, and more satisfying. They assist in building good eating habits, satisfying cravings, and helping you enjoy your meals more. The following are spices I often use in my cooking:

Dry Spices

Sea salt: the more natural, the better – especially the kind produced by evaporation of sea water via exposure to the sun. Sea salt naturally has many good trace elements and minerals. I personally like the variety with added iodine to protect thyroid function. When I was growing up, most people, myself included, developed enlarged thyroids due to a lack of iodine. Once iodine was added to table salt, everyone's thyroid went back to normal size. Hain and Morton are the ones I usually use.

Turmeric: This yellow spice from India can be consumed either in dry powder or raw form. It is anti-inflammatory, cooling in nature, and rich in antioxidant. It assists in neutralizing impaired cells resulting from oxidation, when cells pair up with other good cells, therefore prevents or eases inflammatory conditions within the body. It adds much color and flavor to food as well. I use it in anything from soups to cold dishes, stews, marinating chicken, sautéing vegetables, and stir-fried dishes.

Cumin is very high in antioxidants. Combined with other spices, it is effective in neutralizing free radicals resulting from stress and daily living, thereby easing the aging caused by oxidative stresses. Cumin aids in digestion, detoxifies the liver, cleans up respiratory systems, and enhances immunity. It contains dietary fiber and offers stimulating and antifungal properties as well. It can be incorporated into your daily cooking, either sautéing or baking, or in soups. You don't have to overdo it and overpower the dishes. Simply spice up the dish just right, reaping the benefits of medicine as food and food as medicine while satisfying the taste buds. It is really good on meat barbequed outdoors. You can skewer your meat on sticks and sprinkle on some coarse sea salt, red and black pepper, and cumin. I once took home some restaurant lamb sautéed with hot pepper and cumin and revitalized it with some rice, coconut oil, a bit of sea salt, turmeric, and black and red pepper powder. Now it has become standard practice to add cumin to our stir-fried rice. My then twelve-year-old really loved it. She made it part of her fried rice recipe too.

Cayenne pepper/hot red pepper/paprika: You may be in an imbalanced state, where your energy consumption is higher than the amount of energy your body is making. In other words, you are depleting your body's energy reserves. If so, it may not be a good idea to use these spices often since they irritate the already inflamed yin element in the body. Otherwise these are good spices to add to your meals, giving food zest, stimulating digestion, increasing appetite, and detoxifying the liver. You can make them into a very good morning detoxifier combined with fresh lemon. I love my food spicy, but my Chinese medical friend told me it would benefit me to stay away from it due to my weak yin state stemming from early childhood. I have been gradually building up my energy reserves, so now I am adding these spices to my diet again.

Black pepper: When I was about eight, I had breakouts on my scalp. The fluid spread infection all over, including to my mother, who attempted every possible means to address the infections to no avail. Finally she took some mud from around the core pepper plant, made mud paste by adding water, and applied it to my heavily-infected head. Sure enough, it cured the breakout. Black pepper is actually a very prestigious food across history and cultures. It was once considered an offering for God as well as a measure of a man's wealth. It can be used in any dish, adding some bite and flavor. It is rich in manganese, calcium, iron, vitamin K, and antioxidants, assisting in digestion and elimination, neutralizing oxidation, and protecting the skin.

Cinnamon is one of five spices in powder form (cinnamon, black pepper, cloves, star anise, and fennel) used in almost all Chinese sautés and stews. It can be boiled by wrapping raw cinnamon sticks in a spice bag and adding that to soup base or soups with some beef, chicken, mushrooms, or a combination of these as additional flavoring. Cinnamon is said to promote blood circulation by thinning blood, and has many other medicinal benefits as well as a sweet and pungent flavor. I use it in my nut-apple-date-oatmeal concoction with a dash of brown sugar from plum trees. It tastes so delicious and rich!

Curry is commonly a blend of spices, with turmeric as the main ingredient and others such as black pepper, hot pepper, cumin, cinnamon, and cloves. It is used in dishes of all varieties, and in the yellow mustard often used on hot dogs and hamburgers. Curry has many of the qualities of other dry spices such as assisting in cooling down inflammation, neutralizing the harmful effect of oxidation, and aiding in digestion. It also adds a biting flavor to your foods. Its strong character complements the most compliant foods and enhances the flavor of both dominating and complementing foods, offering much satiety. Like all the different spices, curry aids in keeping your cravings in check, thereby curbing binge eating.

Herbs and Fresh Ingredients

These not only add color, freshness, and taste to any dish, but also offer loads of nutritional benefits as they contain vitamins, minerals, and disease-preventing flavonoids. Look for ways to incorporate them into your meals.

Cilantro detoxifies your system while adding aroma, flavor, and visual appeal to your finished dishes. I use it to finish up practically all my dishes that call for it. Clear soups, with noodles, rice, chicken, beef, or tofu, call for a bit of green and freshness right before serving. You can add it to serving bowls, conserving its freshness, healing power, and nutrients as much as possible.

Garlic is medicinal in whatever way you eat it. It helps with digestion when eaten raw and nourishes when cooked. Even the powdered form can shorten the duration of a cold and ease the severity of symptoms. I especially love the aroma of roasted garlic.

Raw ginger: Ginger is hot or warm in nature. It is considered as ginseng when ingested in the morning, and poison when consumed late in the day. It warms you up on cool or cold days and helps drive out the dampness trapped deep inside the body on hot summer days. My Chinese medical doctor friend told me to drink hot water over raw ginger in the morning. It helps build up immunity, yang energy, and energy reserves. I had some internal flaring when I was in Las Vegas for a trade show one February. When I went back to Chicago's moist air and drank a large cup of water over chrysanthemum, the next day the inflammation was gone. I then made myself a large cup of hot water over ginger and found myself attacked by sneezes. It was my body's innate healing mechanism getting rid of the coldness and dampness accumulated deep down, driven out by the warm properties of ginger. If you are constipated or inflamed with a flaming red tongue and chapped lips, or experience infrequent urination, it might be a good idea to avoid ginger; if you urinate too frequently, a bit of ginger may be a good idea. If you have loose bowels ginger is not a good idea either, because it can irritate the already sensitive digestive system, causing more discomfort.

Basil: This traditional Italian herb is fragrant and fit for use in noodles, soups, and any vegetable dish that calls for the contrasting color and enhancement of flavor. It is especially called for in Italian-style sauces, white or red. I use it in much of my home cooking. I often keep a basil plant on my windowsill facing south, an ideal location for houseplants. Whenever I need a fresh herb to spice up my cooking, I just pick a few leaves, chop them up, and toss them into the food, either as a base flavoring or as a finishing touch.

Green onions/scallions: This family of onions is a variety of fresh flavoring I use quite often during cooking or as a finishing touch for color contrast, flavor, and the added medicinal benefit and nutrition.

Onions of all colors and varieties are said to have cancer-fighting properties. Chop them up really fine, so the compound within can be fully exposed, benefiting the body. They can be eaten raw in salads. Chew very slowly, making sure the saliva is thoroughly mixed in, to fully reap the cancer-fighting benefits. Sautéed onions have a delicious aroma and taste and go very well with many foods as flavoring.

Mushrooms of all varieties are very delicious. They add a meaty flavor, greatly enhancing the richness and satiety of a meal. The three mushrooms that have been researched the most and are believed to boost the immune system while inhibiting tumor growth are shiitake, reishi, and maitake. Even plain white button mushrooms are believed to share some of these benefits. Their healing properties aside, the rich flavors of mushrooms are enough reason to add them to your everyday cooking. You can combine them with garlic, basil, and ginger, or maybe even some fresh turmeric, over a mild flame until tender and soft, then add your main ingredients or combine with soup. Fresh mushrooms can be sautéed right away, while the dried varieties can be ground and used in powder form, soaked, hydrated directly in soups, or boiled as a soup base.

Hot peppers: Fresh hot peppers share some qualities with their dry counterparts. They can be very stimulating, enticing, and delicious when used correctly. They can speed up metabolism and aid in digestion. Hot peppers also provide loads of vitamins such as A, C, K, B6, and folate. If you feel stomach cramps or bellyaches after ingesting hot peppers, shy away from them or ease off the amount you use. Also stay away from them if depletion is on the rise and you feel tired. Ingesting them can cause internal inflammation, with chapped lips and a red, flaming tongue. Hot peppers were a favorite of mine growing up. I was accustomed to having them freshly picked from the fields in spring and summer, sautéed in oil, and sandwiched in between two halves of steamed bread, tasting grassy and earthy. I can hardly find these types of hot peppers now, so I simply stay away from them for the time being.

Nuts and seeds: The most popular ones for cooking are peanuts, pecans, walnuts, and sesame seeds (both white and black). They are full of good oil, vitamins, proteins, and minerals. Nuts can be crushed into small pieces and roasted in oil along with other flavoring spices such as fresh garlic; ginger; turmeric; basil; or red, hot pepper, then combined with main dishes, soup bases, meats, vegetables, or noodles to be further mixed in the cooking process. They add that delicious nutty taste to any dish, turning a somewhat ordinary dish into a celebration.

(f) Be Moderate with Your Portions

Food, like anything, offers the most benefit when it is in the right amount. Overindulging can cause disease from an overstuffed channel in the digestive system. Overeating plays a part in the epidemic of *diabesity* (obesity and diabetes) we are facing in America and in the world. Wealth, or overabundance, as it turns out, is not only a blessing but a responsibility as well, requiring us to make right choices. Our bodies are designed to thrive when they are marginally fed. Humans have starved through most of our two million years of evolution. We have a genetic ability to thrive, not just survive, with a constantly hungry belly. We have never had this much food, and we are not good at digesting this much food as a consequence. We do well with tons of fiber, good fats, and less food than you might think. Just use common sense and be moderate with your portions. Make them big enough to tide you over until the next meal, yet just the right amount to feel comfortable after your meal. If you feel stuffed and uncomfortable, you ate too much food.

Low-starch vegetables should make up 50 to 75 percent of your meal. The balance should be divided between a healthy starch such as a good red potato or a sweet potato, some whole grains, sweet corn, beans, and protein. Protein can come from an animal product or a plant. If it is meat you prefer, the general guideline is the size and thickness of your palm. This will leave you enough room to design your meal per your liking, your bio-individuality, availability, seasons, and special occasions. Of course, the common sense of "stop eating when you are full" applies here. It helps tremendously to take your time and savor your meal.

(g) Make Your Mealtime Sacred

I have often seen people swallowing their food while walking! Some practically inhale their food. It is almost like they swallow the whole plate in an instant. Putting aside the pressure this way of eating puts on your digestive system, what kind of impact does such a meal have on your emotional satiety?

Much love, through the labor and energy of many, has come to your plate, nourishing you as a person – body, mind, heart, and soul. It comes from farmers' endless detailed work day in and day out: preparing the soil, seeding, watering, caring, weeding, and harvesting. If you buy from your local farm stand, this bounty comes to you ready to be cooked. In most cases, your food goes from the farmer's harvest through the usual channels of a transportation company and a wholesale food company, and then to your local store to be made available for purchase. Once it gets to the house, you or someone else in your family pours energy into planning, cleaning, cutting, and cooking. With tremendous love, intention, patience, and nourishing thoughts, the delicious meal is prepared to sit in front of you at the table.

That's not even taking into account the seeds that get the whole process started, or for that matter the soil that has been worked, labored, and sweated over for centuries and the nutrients in it – the oxygen, hydrogen, nitrogen, and all the minerals that have been influenced by the soil's environment including the trees, the air, and the faraway stars. All this is part of your food, in front of you, waiting to be taken in, ingested, and assimilated, thoroughly and completely, into your bloodstream, powering your cells, tissues, bones, muscles, brain, emotions, moods, and being. If you eat animal products, and you are conscious enough or in a position to choose naturally raised animals, you take on the energetics of their natural lives along with the greenness of the pasture and their specific characteristics, nourishing you so you can be the person you are meant to be.

We humans have been trying to outsmart nature, but nature works its wonders in ways that could never be compared to those of a man-made machine or robot. You are responsible for feeding the marvelous creation of nature that is your body; the optimal functioning of its magic is in your hands, controlled by what you put into it. Now let it sink in how sacred this act of eating is. Is it worth your undivided attention? Give it all your attention, with no messaging, no reading, no TV, no arguments, no anger or upsetting emotions – just you and your food, alone or with pleasant companions, good conversation, and loving thoughts.

Food is very transformative. It grows with seeding, good soil, water, and sunshine. In time it is transformed into something nourishing and building, and is absorbed as nutrients by your blood, powering your physical body to be alive and enabling you to live the experiences you are here to live. When you eat with this awareness, you won't just put anything in your precious body anymore. Eating takes on a very different meaning. You want to eat right to help your body help you be the person you are in living the life you yearn to live. It is no longer a chore, but something you do to sustain and enrich your life, in more ways than one. Here are some detailed benefits from this simple act of fully appreciating your meals:

- **First of all,** when you focus on your food and chew slowly, with pleasure, the parasympathetic nerve dominance is initiated, sending hormonal signals that life is in peace and harmony. The bulk of your blood is sent to help digest that food. As you already know, robust digestion is the foundation for robust health, along with all its physical bodily manifestations such as ideal body weight, balanced sugar levels, perfect functioning of body parts, and strong immunity. Some of the underlying stress loses its hold and impact on your body, mind, and heart when you are totally present with your meal, the nourishing source of your physical existence.

- **Second,** when you really enjoy your food, chew your food, taste the flavor, and appreciate its nourishing power, your body's hormonal system has a chance to send you the "full" signal so you can stop eating. We have all had the experience of having our meal interrupted by something we have to do, only to find ourselves full when we return to our food. It takes time for your body to tell you it's full, so it is important to focus on your food at mealtime.

- **Third,** eating mindfully increases satisfaction, satiety, fullness, and richness at all levels. With the simple act of eating your meal, you have eliminated or drastically decreased the chance of binge eating. This alone might be what you need to let go of the extra weight that has been keeping you down. Your body, mind, heart, and soul are so intricately linked that one thing affects the other. Taking the time to enjoy your meal is an important part of living a good and satisfying life. This sacred act of eating goes deep down into you, filling up what has been missing and arousing the emotional memories that are stored in the cells. Some of us experience the association of favorite childhood foods with a warm, fuzzy memory – like the time we spent cooking with our mothers.

- **Fourth,** you might find yourself beginning to choose cleaner meats and cleaner sources for your vegetables. You'll become familiar with your food sources. When you take the source of your nourishment seriously, the chance of wolfing down just anything is much less. The abusive habit of grazing all day long becomes a thing of the past. Your body finally has a chance to really do its wonders: repairing, cleansing, and regenerating. Your immunity is boosted, giving you the edge in fending off all the diseases out there. Always catching the flu when the next person coughs becomes a thing of the past. You might feel yourself catching the flu, but the symptoms are not as severe and don't continue as long. You don't have those miserable nights when your nose is so stuffy that you have to keep your mouth open to breathe, nor will you be waking up in the middle of the night with a horrible, dry pain in your throat from the dry air you are breathing through your open mouth.

- **And fifth,** just by being mindful in the sensual act of eating, you might find excess weight melting away before you even know it. You will be walking around with a glow on your face, contentment in your eyes, and kindness in your words. It is so much easier to be happy when your body is functioning at its best.

(h) Go Easy on White Sugar, White Flour, and Other Refined Carbohydrates

Refined carbohydrates that are quick and easy to ingest are everywhere in our food supply, from pure sugars to refined white flours, white rice, and the majority of packaged foods, in which sugar or flour is the primary ingredient. They quickly jack up your sugar level, causing your body to secrete the hormone insulin, which ushers the excess sugar to cells to store as fat for later use. Due to the lack of fiber in these foods, there is not much mileage for the body to run on, so you crave even more convenient, sugary foods for a quick fix for your lack of energy. You take on more of the same stuff, day in and day out.

Before you know it, you start to develop pre-diabetes or full-blown acute diabetes, when your body becomes insensitive to the insulin floating in the blood, causing excessive amounts of sugars to remain in your bloodstream. Your pancreas secretes more insulin, responding to the situation to assist in the rescue, which does little or nothing due to the resistance of your body. This, in turn, wears out your pancreas, causing you to feel tired all the time. Chronic fatigue becomes your daily reality. The excess blood sugar wreaks havoc in your body, possibly leading to amputation of your hands and legs, causing blindness, and shortening your life span.

This is the epidemic of type II diabetes, or adult onset diabetes. Combined with an overweight condition that is likely to develop, it is the sad phenomenon of diabesity, plaguing the lives of so many Americans and a large proportion of the world population. Just be mindful about your food intake. When you cook at home, be sure to limit your use of sugars, flours, and refined carbohydrates, and use healthier, more wholesome and natural substitutes.

For sugar, you can always substitute raw honey, which has very good healing properties. Real maple syrup is better than refined white sugar as well, as are many other sugars that are less processed, such as plum tree sugar, rock sugar, coconut sugar, and sugar cane. Watch out for high fructose corn syrup. It seems to mess up the hormonal system's hunger and fullness signaling, causing you to overeat. Even though all these natural sugars still have glucose, they are loaded with minerals and vitamins. The key is always moderation. Overconsumption of anything, regardless of what it is, causes harm to the body and triggers stress in the digestive system. Avoid artificial sweeteners and sugar replacements. They are nothing but toxic chemicals. Most of the beet sugar out there is genetically modified; stay away from this as well. If you are going to have a sweet, be sure it is the real thing.

(i) Avoid Packaged Foods

It is said that the average American consumes about ten pounds of sugar per year, most of which comes from sugars hidden in packaged foods and sugary drinks. Many of us think we are not consuming sugar at all even though we ingest these foods. If you eat packaged foods and drink soft drinks, you are taking in tons of sugar. The American Diabetes Association says that about 29.1 million Americans, or 9.3 percent of the population, suffer from diabetes (2012 statistics, 2014 report), of which 8.1 million are undiagnosed; and that 86 million Americans aged twenty and over are pre-diabetic. It is predicted that ten years down the road, the majority of Americans will have diabetes or pre-diabetes.

Many of the packaged foods on the market are man-made stuff – a far cry from real food. To top it off, they are loaded with preservatives, dyes, and all sorts of flavor enhancers to keep you wanting more. That does not even take into account the chemicals, pesticides, genetically modified organisms (GMOs), antibiotics, and heaps of sugar and salt they are loaded with. If you have to purchase packaged goods, read the ingredients list. At least be sure that the first ingredient is the food it claims to be. If the first ingredient is sugar, ditch it. If the list has more than five ingredients, with many hard to pronounce, put it back on the shelf.

(j) Bio-Individuality

As humans, we all share the traits of eating, sleeping, drinking, moving around, thinking, feeling, and being. Yet the way we do each is different. You are biologically different from the person next to you. In the whole history of mankind over millions of years of evolution, you are the only one .. your skin, with your unique digestive tract, your build, your thumbprint, the way you think, the way you speak, the way you express yourself, the way you digest your food, and the way you assimilate your emotions. There is not another person who is your exact duplicate. One person's food can very well be another's poison.

This is proof enough as to why there are so many diet theories out there encouraging weight loss through polar opposite approaches. Yet the promoters enthusiastically and passionately sing the numerous benefits and wonders of their diets. Many people follow a diet to the letter, lose the weight, seemingly get better, and then gain it all back.

Dr. Peter D'Adamo, author of *Eat Right for Your Type: The Individualized Diet Solution to Staying Healthy, Living Longer & Achieving Your Ideal Weight*, promotes the idea that people with different blood types thrive on different foods. This concept is well known in China and Japan. It says that those with blood type A are natural vegetarians, those with type O are meat-eaters, and those with types B and AB fall somewhere in between. This seems to apply to many of the people I know. I have blood type A, and I love more vegetables than meat and experience better elimination and digestion when I eat vegetables. I feel lighter in general as well, even though I do love to include small amounts of clean animal protein in my meals, including various meats and eggs.

I remember hearing raw-food enthusiasts passionately speaking about raw foods and their amazing benefits when I was at the Health Coach Training Program at IIN. I was so impressed that I started incorporating more raw foods into my meals – more salads than ever. It was winter, and bitterly cold, and soon afterward I found myself shivering quite a bit. At that time I had a neighbor who consumed raw foods on a daily basis. They seemed to work for her even in the winter. By the way, she looks fifty, while her chronological age is over seventy. When I asked her whether she was feeling cold or not, she replied that she just turned the heat high in her house, which seems to go against the grain of nature to me. Then again, I am not her. I gradually added salads and certain raw foods back into my meals, especially more so in summer.

It is very interesting that IIN teaches students every diet under the sun. Halfway through the program, most of us did not know what to eat anymore. We were being forced to think on our own, to come up with ideas that work the best for us and our clients. A diet that suits you is one that works with your biology, lifestyle, level of activity, ethnicity, upbringing, the season, the time of day, and the different phases of your life. The curriculum at IIN was designed so we would learn to consult our bodies and listen to their innate wisdom.

For a little while I experimented with cooking quinoa for breakfast. The popularity of this grain has shot through the roof due to the fact that it grows on the high plains of the Andes of South America. Quinoa has an inherent tolerance for dry conditions to the point that when it gets too dry, it just stops growing until it rains. After consuming this grain a couple of mornings, my old condition of having a blister in the left corner of my mouth returned. It indicated an internally flared state, which diminished right away after I eased off my consumption of quinoa. Often the very quality of your food is what causes you to have certain conditions in your body or brings out certain imbalances.

So start to get intimate with your body. Listen to its needs and wants and what it thrives on. What makes it tired? What triggers gassy conditions? What gives you energy? What makes your heart sing? What makes your soul light? What makes your steps springy? What feeds your cravings? It is all about embracing your individuality in every aspect of your life. You know that you can't really fool yourself, because your body will let you know it.

It is only when you totally face your individuality that you start to flourish. This includes embracing your uniqueness in all areas of your life, such as the food that nourishes you as a person, the lifestyle that honors you as the unique individual you are, and the things you do to fully express your purpose in this lifetime. Once you experience this natural high, you will never, never, never want to live the kind of life you led before, with boredom, tiredness, and stress as your perceived reality. You will want to do that which feeds your bio-individuality.

(k) The 90/10 Rule

I often hear people say they feel bad because they have eaten something sweet, messing up their resolve to not eat anything bad. That is what happens with many of the strict diets out there as well. They seem very good at first, but the challenge is that people can't stick to them. Once the binge eating starts, it is hard to stop. A diet built on will power is very challenging to sustain when a craving kicks in with its deeply rooted life force. All too often will power gives in to an unyielding craving that has a life of its own. You might find yourself eating the very thing you are trying to avoid. Moreover, denying yourself the very foods your body craves leaves you feeling unsatisfied and deprived. You will break free from your will power at some point when you least expect it.

The golden rule is to eat what is good for your body, mind, heart, and soul 90 percent of the time. The other 10 percent of the time, eat according to your impulses. You can adjust your percentage based on your circumstances; maybe 80/20 works better for you. Chances are once you are on a solid path of healthy and deeply satisfying eating, you won't have many cravings for anything else. But if you do, embrace them. Make sure you understand them for what they are and don't make a habit of giving in every time. The key is to keep your supporting habit strong, making it the main theme.

Look for the healthier version of whatever you are craving. Whatever improvements you make, you are benefiting your body in building up. For example, you can make pizza at home with freshly-made dough using almond flour, sweet potato flour, or mung bean flour. If you make the dough with refined white flour, make it thin. Use good, clean, organic meat from naturally raised animals. Buy clean, organic, locally-grown vegetables. Better yet, pick vegetables from your own garden. Choose organic cheese from naturally raised cows fed with organic feeds, free from growth hormones, GMOs, and all other added chemicals. You can eat pizza as long as you have this awareness and a love of cooking healthy, and you will be just fine. Chances are once you are feeding your body wholesome, building, nourishing fuel, it will crave whole, simple foods.

Chapter Nine

Make Your Kitchen the Center of Nourishment and Healing

I grew up with my mother constantly cooking in the kitchen, and I helped her with whatever I could. Either it was rolling dough, pushing the firing device, cutting vegetables, picking or cleaning vegetables, or just simply hanging with her. The whole family, even guests when we had some, often stayed in the kitchen, talking about either food or life in general. Kitchen, food, and life were intricately linked together.

Sampling was one of the perks during our cooking. Cooking and food: the creation, the ease, the joy, the peace, and the satisfaction are all part of this cozy memory. When I first came to America, I was studying the MBA program at the University of Massachusetts Dartmouth. With all the information management systems, the statistical analysis, and the accounting and marketing courses, I was having a very trying time, having been an English major back in college in China. One day a friend of mine I invited for dinner commented that when I was cooking I looked truly happy and relaxed and seemed to know what I was doing.

These days, regardless of how busy I am, I almost always enjoy putting something together quickly – something nourishing, delicious, and relatively easy to make, good for the body and the wallet, from whatever ingredients I have in the pantry or the refrigerator. The very act of cooking connects me with my center, sort of like a form of meditation, where I can simply act from intuition and innate knowing. Needless to say, I had strayed away from this tradition for a while, being swept into the fast lane of fast food and declining health.

Sometimes I can't help but think that if there had been a Burger King or McDonald's back when I was growing up, people would most likely have eaten that, and would most likely have gotten big and unhealthy. And this is just what has been happening in China since fast food chains established a presence in all the major cities. Large numbers of people are showing signs of diabetes, and China ranks number two in the world, right after India. And what if there had been abundant supplies of beef, chicken, and pork? Would my mother have cooked tons of that? I remember when things got better in China, one of my older brothers commented that he got nauseated from eating too much pork. I have never been much of a meat eater, as it did not sit well with me either. I have always gravitated towards more vegetables. On my healing journey I gained the understanding and awareness of why I behaved the way I did growing up, and in America merging in. I was just being carried along by the strong circumstantial tide without much understanding and awareness about food, health, well-being, and the effect they had on my body and mind.

In a broad sense, this is what has been happening in America: The majority of Americans have been buying ready-made or semi-ready-made food from restaurants and supermarkets, allowing the big food business free reign in cooking our food for us. I was puzzled at first as to why anyone would want to buy a prepared salad from the supermarket, until I became a part of the herd. As a by-product or wake-up call, my body broke down. I was not too surprised when my doctor told me my cholesterol level was on the high end and that I needed to be careful. No instructions were given as to how to go about being careful.

Diabesity – the combination of obesity and diabetes – a condition brought to my awareness during my IIN study, affects one billion people worldwide, including one hundred million Americans, and the trend is on the rise. It is believed to be the major cause of heart disease, stroke, dementia, cancer, kidney failure, and blindness. A big contributing factor in diabesity is leaving our food preparation to corporate food giants whose main interest is the bottom line. Coming from a way of life where everything was done from scratch, I was surprised to see the poor kitchen skills of most Americans, skills that came to me naturally.

Your kitchen can become the center of attention in your family, where your whole family, including guests, participate in the cooking. As you cook, you can interact and hold conversations. In the process of cooking and eating, you not only create something delicious and nutritious but something that feeds your mind, body, heart, and soul. You also build a tradition of a rich life with the aromas, deliciousness, spices, and flavors, all of which are stored in your cells as memories. If you have young kids, that tradition will be part of their heritage, benefiting them in astonishing ways.

When corporations cook your food, you leave yourself open to the whole nine yards of industrial downfalls in your food, things like pesticides, hormones, and GMOs. You are exposed to all sorts of inferior-quality ingredients as well as all the chemical flavor-enhancers and other additives that make you crave these foods. There is also the factor of preparation method, such as deep frying, which can result in cancer-causing compounds. The seemingly healthy vegetable oils used in packaged foods can be harmful, too, if they come from genetically modified soybeans, corn, or cottonseeds. This is very likely given the fact that about 90 percent of such crops are genetically modified. This goes for restaurant cooking as well. And cooking at home cannot guarantee the healthiest meal if you unconsciously buy ingredients without understanding and paying attention to their sources.

The more you cook at home with mindfully selected ingredients, the more you and your family will enjoy home-cooked meals that are loaded with love, cost less, taste better, and are healthier. Let's face it, you need to eat. You are what you eat and assimilate. It makes perfect sense to make cooking part of life and cook as often as you can. It will definitely help you avoid most of the industrial toxins in food, the degree of which is dependent on the degree to which you take charge of your own food intake.

Cooking can be a great way to express your creativity and relax into the act of doing something that flows from deep within. With practice, it can be the very thing you need to reconnect with your deeper self, immersing in the creation that is the expression of your soul, mingled with color, texture, aroma, and taste. It can be deeply satisfying and gratifying to the body, mind, heart, and soul. It will also save you tons of money compared to eating similar-quality foods at restaurants. Here is what you can do to get started if you are not doing so already:

1. Shop For and Store Basic Ingredients

Start shopping for healthy basic ingredients and store them in your kitchen. Eat your way to health and happiness.

Dry spices: Buy the dry spices mentioned earlier, preferably in organic form to get the most nutritional value and avoid potential health risks caused by irradiation in food processing. Small jars are better than big jars, since spices are better fresh than aged. Transfer loose spices into small, clean, washed jars with tight lids for safe storage. Store them in cool, dark places to prevent oxidative damage from light and oxygen.

Fresh herbs have more flavor than their dried versions, so shoot for fresh whenever you can. Many are readily available in a variety of stores. Most can be wrapped and stored in the refrigerator. Ginger and turmeric are best kept frozen. Simply cut them up into smaller chunks, wrap in plastic bags, and store in the freezer. They can be used on an as-needed basis. Lemons can be stored either refrigerated or frozen. Garlic and onions can be stored in your pantry in wooden containers or paper bags.

Vegetables and fruits:

- If you can, shop local, from a farm stand or a farmer's market, when in season, for maximum freshness, nutrients, sustainability, safety, and nourishing value. Local markets and farmer's markets normally carry produce from small farms where farmers use small sprayers to treat bugs and weeds, thereby leaving less chemical residue on produce. Ethnic stores normally carry items not widely consumed that are most likely farmed by small farmers as well, due to the scale of production. Thoroughly wash your produce. When I wash vegetables bought in Chinatown, I often see bugs feeding on the leafy greens even after they have been in the refrigerator for a couple of days.

- When making choices between locally grown produce and organics imported from overseas, I normally pick the local versions because they are fresher straight from the farm to my kitchen, and they carry local elements that better support me as the eater I am – body, mind, heart, and soul.

- In winter, when there are fewer choices, shop at your local market. Use the food scores published by the Environmental Working Group (EWG) and buy their "Clean 15," which are the fifteen fruits and vegetables that contain the fewest amounts of pesticide residue through traditional means of production. For 2015, they were the following:

avocado
sweet corn (non-GMO variety)
pineapple
cabbage
sweet peas (frozen)
onion
asparagus
mango
papaya
kiwi
eggplant
grapefruit
cantaloupe
cauliflower
sweet potato

- Watch for EWG's "Dirty Dozen" and "Dirty Dozen Plus" (plus two), and go organic if you can afford to; otherwise eat organic until they become available locally at harvest time, or make sure to cook them, since "pesticide levels typically diminish when food is cooked," according to EWG. This will keep you safe while stretching your dollar. Here is EWG's 2015 Dirty Dozen, in descending order of danger:

  1. Apples
  2. Peaches
  3. Nectarines
  4. Strawberries
  5. Grapes
  6. Celery

7. Spinach
8. Sweet bell peppers
9. Cucumbers
10. Cherry tomatoes
11. Snap peas – imported
12. Potatoes

- Keep in mind that most of the popular everyday foods such as potatoes and tomatoes are mass-produced, where industrial strength sprayers are normally used to treat bugs and kill weeds. This exposes these foods to heavy doses of chemicals. It is very wise to follow EWG's guidance in regard to residue levels in this produce.

Grains: These can be bought at your local market, a health food market like WholeFoods, or an ethnic market. Buy them in season and store them in airtight containers in cool places. Buy those that have not been processed or treated with any anti-bug substances. Be aware that anything bugs won't touch won't be able to feed the healthy bugs living in your gut that assist in digesting food and keeping your immunity strong. Aim for grains with their outer layer, bran, and endosperm kept intact – whole grains.

Legumes and beans: Store them in tight bags or jars, in easy-to-access cooler places. Again, buy a small quantity to keep your supply fresh.

2. Cooking Basics

Cooking does not need to be fancy and complicated. As a matter of fact, if you are cooking daily already, it might be second nature to you. If you have hardly ever cooked, get started. Very soon you will be rewarded by the creations of your own labor. You might even find yourself enjoying it, unleashing some of your creative potential you never knew existed.

Cooking is not rocket science. It is pretty much intuitive once you get the hang of it. I create meals from memory based on the aroma and the way the food looks, from cookbooks, from watching cooking on TV, or from watching friends cook their recipes. You can follow recipes if you like, especially if you are experimenting with something new. Once you do this for a while, you will be able to come up with your own creations fanned by your own imagination, insight, taste buds, and cravings. In your kitchen, you are the king or queen, and the sky is the limit! It's a great idea to get your family involved, all becoming part of the learning, creating, and harmonious, happy living process.

If you are very new to cooking, here is a quick summary of the various common cooking methods:

- **Boiling** is just as what it sounds like. Boil your food in bubbling water, completely or partially immersed, so that the food absorbs the water into its cell walls while the minerals from the food leak into the water. The leftover water is a good soup base if the food is relatively clean.

- **Steaming** is using the steam from simmering water to cook the food, the same idea as steaming in a hot sauna. Use a steamer for this, which is a perforated platform that holds the food above the water, or any type of platform that does the same thing. Start with cold water, put the food on top of the steamer over the water, cover, bring to a boil or until steam is coming out from all sides of the lid, and reduce the heat to low, simmering until the food is cooked but still crisp. Steaming preserves more of the minerals in the food by allowing it to absorb the rising moisture in the closed environment of the cooking device.

- **Sautéing, stir-frying, and pan-frying** are all dry heating methods that don't use water. Use just enough cooking oil to quickly sear the food and lock the nutrients in. During the process, some water might come out of the food, causing it to wilt. For most foods it's best to stop cooking just before this occurs to retain a crisp texture.

- **Baking and grilling** are done in the oven. Baking applies even heat to the entire dish and is usually a long-term process, while grilling applies direct heat or flame to the surface of the food and is a faster method of cooking, such as for steaks and fish.

You can use any of the methods, or a combination of several, for your cooking.

3. Wholesome and Delicious Dishes

Vegetable Dishes

Salads: It is always good to incorporate tons of fresh salads in your meals, especially in spring and summer. They are quick to prepare and add fiber, flavor, and nutrients to your daily routine, perfect for raising the nutritional value of any given meal. Wash your green ingredients and pat or spin dry if possible – watery greens make for a soggy salad. If they are non-organic, wash once with water, then use some diluted vinegar to wash them again, then rinse off. My house salad could be anything, whatever I have on hand: some leafy greens and iceberg lettuce mixed with chopped celery, grated carrots, white or sweet onions, cucumbers, and tomatoes. Add finely chopped garlic for that fresh garlic taste, fresh-squeezed lemon juice or good vinegar, olive oil, maybe even some sesame oil for a nutty flavor, sea salt, pepper, and turmeric to taste. I always love some nuts in the mix as well. You can add fruit such as organic strawberries, apples, or blueberries to your salad. For a simple salad, just wash off some leafy vegetable mix and serve as a side dish.

Sautéed leafy greens: Wash them thoroughly, break them with your hands into bite-sized pieces, or have your kids do it. Chop up some garlic, raw ginger, or raw turmeric if you have some. Heat up a sauté pan or wok over medium heat (I always use a flat ceramic pan), using about a tablespoon of coconut oil or some other healthy cooking oil. Once the oil melts or is heated, put your raw spices in – the garlic, ginger, turmeric. Stir with a wooden spoon, or just a pair of chopsticks until an aroma arises. Then put in your leafy greens, stir a bit, and spice them with pinches of sea salt, black pepper, red pepper or cayenne pepper, and powdered turmeric if you don't have the raw form, "to taste," which means taste the dish and stop when the level of flavor is what you prefer. Start with less, especially the salt. Once it is in, you can't take it out if it is too salty, and you can always add more if it is not salty enough. Once the greens are wilted, they should be done – about five minutes. Use your judgment here. Some people prefer them quite limp, and some like them half-cooked, with a bite of crunchiness and optimum vitamin retention, yet enough to destroy most bacteria and pesticides and assist with digestion. Serve them as a side dish in a big, colorful serving bowl for a contrast of colors.

Quick stir-fried vegetables: Heat up a sauté pan or wok over medium heat, using about a tablespoon of coconut oil or some other healthy cooking oil. Once the oil melts or is heated, put your raw spices in – garlic, ginger, turmeric. Stir until an aroma arises. I normally add some mushrooms and sliced onions right after the raw spices or as raw spices. They add so much aroma and flavor to the dish, making it more appetizing. There is quite a collection of vegetables that can be cooked this way, yielding something delicious and nutritious with zest, flavor, and texture. They include all varieties of peppers in various colors: red, yellow, green, purple; and onions of all colors: red, white, and yellow. Celery and broccoli can be cooked this way as well, but due to their low water content, add a bit of water to the pan after they've been stirred a bit and they're coated with oil. Vegetables take a couple minutes longer than greens.

Green beans and other vegetables that take longer to cook: Clean the vegetables. For green beans, snap the two ends off with your hands, as well as the strings on either side that come off with the ends, and break them in half. Beat up two cloves of garlic with the side of your heavy cutting knife. You can also use some raw ginger and raw turmeric if you like. Cut them into very fine pieces. Heat up a sauté pan or wok over medium heat, using about a tablespoon of coconut oil or some other healthy cooking oil. Once the oil melts or is heated, put your raw spices in – garlic, ginger, turmeric. Stir until an aroma arises. Then add the prepared green beans, stirring quickly. Spice with a pinch of sea salt, black pepper, red pepper or cayenne pepper, and turmeric, to taste. Sprinkle a bit of cold water over the spice so it can be thoroughly mixed in with the vegetables. Once the green beans turn bright green, turn down the fire to a minimum. Simmer for about 10 minutes. Make sure there is enough liquid in the bottom of the pan to prevent burning (about a quarter cup of water).

This is how I learned to cook green beans in America. They take much longer to cook than the variety I was accustomed to when I was in China. When I first cooked green beans in America, I cooked them the same way I had in China: sautéed over medium heat; as soon as the color turned, the fire was turned off and the dish was considered done. But my green beans came out raw. Since then I have added simmering time for doneness and the maximum amount of nutritional value with a combination of a short time over high heat and a longer time over low heat. I serve my green bean dish at family gatherings, at neighborhood parties, and at the many Chinese New Year celebrations with neighbors, friends, and clients. It has been a favorite every single time. It is so popular that I get phone calls from neighbors when guests show up, asking me how to prepare the dish at the last minute. People often see me buying heaps of green beans at the store and stop to ask me how to cook them. My daughter often asks me to cook green beans this way to serve as a side dish when we have chicken, salmon, or any other meal.

Cauliflower, Brussels sprouts, zucchini, yellow squash, and red carrots can be cooked the same way, cut into big chunks, most requiring longer cooking times for a bit more softening.

White potatoes sautéed with vinegar: Vinegar added at the right time gives vegetables a crunchy texture. Wash three or four medium-sized potatoes, remove the eyes and green parts (poisonous according to Chinese tradition), shred or slice thinly, whichever way you prefer, either by hand or using a food processor. Because of the heavy starch content in potatoes, put the pieces in a large bowl filled with water. Rinse out the starchy content a few times, the same way you do rice. Keep changing the water until it becomes clear. This only takes a few seconds. Keep your potatoes fully immersed, waiting in the big bowl of water, ready to be sautéed (the color changes to dark if exposed to air). You can use any of the following as enhancers for an appetizing color, taste, or texture:

- One small stalk of celery, sliced
- One small carrot, sliced or shredded to match the cut of your potatoes
- One green scallion, thinly sliced
- One dry red pepper or one or two hot green peppers – jalapeno is okay (if you are up to the spiciness), in thin slices or shreds

Use the same sautéing method as in the above recipes, using a sauté pan with some oil over medium heat. Stir in the spices – garlic, ginger, and turmeric – and add the red or green peppers. When the aroma rises, fish out the potatoes from the bowl with your hands and put them in the sizzling pan. If some water is mixed in, it is perfectly okay, since that will help with the moisture content in the mix. While potatoes are cooking, they will absorb the extra moisture due to their starchy content. Add your celery and/or carrot if you like. Flip the vegetables a few times with a wooden flipper. Then stir in a tablespoon of vinegar, which adds crunchiness to the dish, preventing it from becoming a pile of mush. You can also sprinkle in about a tablespoon of cooking wine if you like; the alcohol will evaporate during cooking, leaving the wine flavor. They normally will take about five minutes to cook once the vinegar is in. Add dry spices such as sea salt, black or cayenne pepper, and turmeric. Test for doneness and cook until you like the consistency. Turn off the fire and place in a serving dish. Garnish with the sliced scallion by sprinkling the slices on top.

Lotus root sautéed with vinegar: This is another dish that can be cooked in the same manner. Lotus root is a Chinese root vegetable. It grows under water with pretty flowers floating on the surface in spring. This was a novelty food used during the New Year's season for entertaining guests or for celebrations of any sort when I was growing up. The lotus flower is a symbol of awakening in Eastern culture, with layers of beautiful petals opening out from the middle. Lotus root can be bought in Chinatown. My family jokes about it every time when we have lotus root, saying we are living it up, being the rich and the royal.

Chinese cabbage sautéed with vinegar: Chinese cabbage or regular cabbage can be cooked in the same way, with or without the celery, carrot, and scallion.

Root vegetables are harvested in the fall and best eaten in winter. They are warming, sustaining, building, and grounding. They entrench deep down in the earth, taking up all the nutrients from the soil. They contain phytonutrients absorbed from the sun through the leaves above ground, and have a starchy, nourishing quality. The best way to cook them is stewing. Quickly sauté your ginger, garlic, and turmeric in heated oil , add the cubed root vegetables, and then some water, and simmer over low heat.

They can be simmered with beef as a stew as well. They enhance the beefy flavor and color without competing or overpowering it. Napa cabbage, carrots, and potatoes go beautifully in a beef stew. Beets are best cooked by themselves.

Here is how to get your food stewing:

- Small bits of raw ginger and turmeric
- Mashed garlic
- Cubed vegetables, ready to be used
- One dried red pepper or hot green pepper, chopped – optional if you like your stew to have some bite
- Chopped scallions and/or cilantro

Use a big saucepan to heat up a generous amount of oil or ghee over medium heat. Stir in the spices, then the vegetables and peppers. Quickly stir a few times. Spice using your favorite dry spices. Pour in a half cup of water. Then turn the fire to low and simmer for about half an hour, or until done to your taste. Scoop up into a serving dish and sprinkle your chopped scallion and/or cilantro over the dish to garnish, adding color, freshness, appeal, and nutritional value.

Eggplant: This dish is also popular with my guests. Even my Chinese community loves it. I started making it in the early 1980s when I was in college back in Xian, China. It was a dish I liked from the student restaurant. I experimented making it when I went back home for winter vacation. My mother was so proud of me, telling everyone how good my eggplant was! So let's get to it:

- One egg
- Two tablespoons flour
- Sea salt and pepper, both black and red (cayenne pepper or paprika)
- Turmeric
- One small jar of coconut oil or other good cooking oils mentioned earlier
- One medium eggplant, cut into rectangular shapes, a half-inch thick and two to three inches long
- A large clove of garlic, or two small ones, finely chopped
- One large or two medium-sized tomatoes cubed into small pieces
- A few drops of sesame oil, for taste
- A few fresh cilantro sprigs, loosely broken into long pieces for garnishing
- Half a thinly shredded scallion, both white and green parts, for garnishing

Eggplants soak up oil like a sponge, so you can either use more good oil or presoak the freshly cut eggplant in water for about one hour, which reduces the absorption of oil. I prefer loads of oil in this dish, rich with delicious and meaty flavor.

In a soup bowl, break the egg. Stir well. Then mix in the flour and pinches of sea salt, peppers, paprika, and turmeric. Add a quarter cup of water and mix well. Heat up a flat saucepan and melt a generous amount of coconut oil or other oil. Completely cover the inside bottom of the pan with oil, then some more. Use medium to low heat to prevent the oil from smoking. Carefully dip each piece of eggplant in the egg batter. Then put it in the saucepan. Be sure each makes contact with the bottom and oil. Cook a few at a time, flipping them often. Turn them when the bottom sides are browned and wilted. Once all sides are browned, soft, and cooked, fish the pieces out and place them on a plate, ready for the final step. If the bottom of the pan dries out, add more oil to it. Repeat the process with all the eggplant pieces until all are done. Then rinse out the pan for the final mixing stage.

Heat up a wok or a large saucepan over medium heat, adding a bit of cooking oil just to keep the food from sticking. Put in the chopped garlic. Once the aroma rises, put in the diced tomato. Spice it up with a bit of sea salt, black and red pepper/cayenne pepper, or paprika. Stir constantly until the tomato is cooked down, about five minutes. Then put in the cooked eggplant. Flip with a flat flipper a few times, preserving the shape of the eggplant as much as you can. Then turn off the fire. Carefully scoop up the cooked content into a serving dish. Sprinkle with a few drops of sesame oil. Garnish with the loose cilantro and scallion.

Fermented vegetables: My mom always made a few large jars of fermented vegetables to tide us over the winter. The vegetables were normally the late fall harvest, such as Chinese radish/daikon radish, carrots, and Chinese mustard greens. It was a very common scene when right after the harvest the whole village would be making fermented Chinese radish. Women were busy boiling water and washing and trimming the vegetables. The men helped clean out large heavy ceramic jars of various sizes, some as large as three feet high, round with smaller bases and openings. The common practice was that once the jar was cleaned out, a layer of salt would be laid on the bottom, then a layer of the whole trimmed radish would be added, then another layer of salt over that, then the radish, then salt, radish, salt, radish, salt. You keep going until the jar is about 80 percent full.

Cinnamon sticks, raw peppercorns, peeled whole garlic cloves, long red hot peppers, raw ginger, or whole cloves were often added in the layering step as well, for added flavor. Then cooled boiled water was poured into the jar, so that all the vegetables were immersed underneath the water, then a few inches more. Then a straw cover was laid over the opening of the jar, with a ceramic cover over that to keep it tight enough yet breathing. It was stored in a dark place for a few months for when the winter months kicked in and fresh vegetables were scarce.

I can see it in my mind's eye… my mom fishing out one large, long radish from the jar. It would be finely shredded, along with some finely sliced green onion that had been buried in dirt and covered with corn yards (or corn sticks – from the plant stems) or simply placed in the dirt where it normally grew. Then she would heat up some hot oil in a ladle with a long handle over the fire in the cooking pit, and pour it over the onion and radish.

This fermentation process used way more salt than what is being recommended in some of the fermentation recipes out there these days. The common name for that style of fermented vegetables is salty vegetables. Yet there was no illness known to be associated with that. Fermented radish was only served with food that was simple and free of salt or other spices, such as morning porridges and steamed bread, and in small portions like a condiment. It was hardly ever served with flavorful foods such as noodles with vegetables. We didn't eat it for the benefit of introducing more gut bacteria; it was made so there would be vegetables for the long winter months, though some other methods were employed to preserve vegetables such as burying them in the dirt outside in the open and cold.

During my IIN Health Coach Training Program, I heard quite a few people talking about gut bacteria and fermented foods and their many healing properties. I was amazed as to the wisdom of the lifestyle I was brought up with, as we weren't aware of its simplicity, beauty, and health-related benefits. For a while, after my weight, blood sugar, and mental clarity had been brought to a healthy state, I still struggled with a low energy level. I heard probiotic pioneer Natasha Treven talking about her probiotics on the radio and how many of the benefits would address my symptoms of bloating and tiredness. I ordered some, and they worked wonders. Once my daughter's dad complained to me about how bloated he was and asked me if there was something he could eat to ease up that condition since the probiotics had run out at that time. It occurred to me that I could experiment with fermented vegetables.

All I did that first time was cut up some cabbages I had in the fridge and rub them with salt, garlic, turmeric, and black pepper in a big ceramic bowl. Then I stuffed the mixture into a big, clean, used pickle jar, with a little splash of water on top. A few hours later, before bedtime, he ate some of the vegetables, and told me the next day that he was feeling better and the bloating had eased off. In about a week that jar of vegetables was gone, before they even had enough time to properly ferment. I stopped ordering the probiotics and since then have been consuming my fermented vegetables of various varieties, in addition to some Chinese herbs.

Lacto-fermentation is a traditional fermentation process in which starches and sugars in vegetables and fruits transform to lactic acid through a friendly bacterium known as lactobacilli. Not only does it help preserve the freshness and nutrients in the food due to no heat being used, but it also reinforces gut bacteria function by providing nutrition, flora, fiber, ease of digestion, and flavor. It is estimated that humans carry about *100 trillion microorganisms* (gut bacteria) in our intestines – *ten times more than the total number of cells in our bodies.* Many factors affect whether this population thrives or diminishes, and it obviously performs an important role in the proper functioning of the host body. Some documented functions are: assisting the body in utilizing some of the undigested carbohydrates it consumes; producing and facilitating the body's absorption of essential vitamins like vitamin K; impacting the gut and systemic immune system in a continuous and dynamic way; playing a major role in metabolizing carcinogens that naturally occur during cooking, especially over high heat, therefore helping in the prevention of tumors; and preventing allergies – overreactions of the immune system to non-harmful antigens – and inflammatory bowel disease.

Experiment and get started. The key elements in natural fermentation are the right proportion of salt and the right temperature – starting off at about 70°F and then reducing the temperature to 50° to 60° for the flavor and culture to settle in; an oxygen-free environment; and darkness for fermenting and storage.

Many vegetables ferment nicely, such as cabbages, daikon radish, cucumbers, any sort of greens with long stems, carrots, mushrooms, garlic, cauliflower, and white and purple radishes. Onions, tomatoes, celeries, and hot peppers are good complements for fermentation with other vegetables. I always love the mixture of colors and vegetables.

Suggested ingredients:

- A blend of herbs or any one you prefer, fresh or dried whole, half to one teaspoon each: peppercorns, caraway seed, mustard seed, coriander; or one bay leaf (optional)
- Two pounds of vegetables, washed and cut, any one or a mixed batch of the above will do
- About three tablespoons of salt (most recipes suggest two tablespoons, but it can be a little more if it is coarse

sea salt; stick with salt without iodine – coarse sea salt provides more flavor and minerals)

- A large pickle jar that holds about 80 fluid ounces, or two smaller ones, cleaned and dried
- Two cloves of garlic, coarsely chopped
- A few stems of dill, broken into short pieces
- Other complementary vegetables such as a little bit of sliced onion, hot pepper, or mushrooms (optional)
- About two cups of non-chlorinated tap water or cooled boiled chlorinated tap water (boil at least ten minutes)

Add any of the dry herbs to four cups of water, if it's a small batch, and bring to a boil over medium-high heat. Simmer for about half an hour for the flavors to disperse into the water, and let this cool while you wash and cut the vegetables and salt them thoroughly using your hands to rub the salt in.

When the water is cool, transfer the vegetables to the cleaned jar or jars with fresh garlic, dill, and hot pepper on top. Pour the prepared water into the jar so that the vegetables are completely immersed in the water, then add an additional inch of water to create an oxygen-free environment. Make sure all the vegetables are underneath the water, otherwise exposure to the air will create mildew. If discoloring or mildew occurs, discard any infected vegetables. You can place something heavy over the vegetables to weigh them down, but so far I haven't had to do that; all I do is to constantly push the vegetables down any time I see them being exposed to air. I always make sure to discard any part that doesn't look healthy. Cover loosely with the lid, leaving some space for the gas (carbon dioxide) that is given off in the fermenting process to escape. Built-up gas can make the jar explode if it's covered too tightly.

The presence of oxygen can produce yeast appearing as white, fuzzy balls on top of the water. Remove them every week or so. They are harmless, but not pleasant to the taste buds. My mother's fermentation jars had some of these fuzzy balls when the weather got warmer, as well as some boneless bugs swimming around. My mom just calmly pushed them out of the way, fished out her fermented daikon radish, rinsed it in clean water, and proceeded as usual. Anything bugs eat is good for the bugs residing in your gut. Nevertheless, let's not get carried away here; if you see bugs, remove them or dump the whole thing if the idea doesn't sit well with you.

Place the jar on a low counter where the temperature is more stable, away from windows and exposure to heat and sun for a couple of days. Then move it to a cooler place such as an unheated basement or put it in the refrigerator for further fermentation for a couple of weeks. Proper fermentation ensures that enough lactic acid is produced for the intended benefits. Aged fermentation tastes better, too – when the daikon radish turns a golden yellow.

Experiment with the amount of salt until you have obtained the ideal taste – salty enough to preserve the vegetables yet light enough to be enjoyable, crunchy, and fresh to the bite. Several times I spread more salt in the top of the jar, and loved the aged fermentation with the saltier flavor. With a heavier dose of salt, at least three weeks of fermentation is needed for the salt to set in. You can also increase the other flavoring ingredients by about one spoonful if you like more flavor.

You can fish out just enough for one meal at a time – a condiment-sized serving to go along with your main dishes. It takes some trial and error to get just the right combination. It helps to start small, maybe one-half to one pound of vegetables, until you get the hang of it. It benefits the bugs in your gut, and therefore your health. It is good for your wallet, too. Have fun experimenting.

Chinese Tofu: I grew up watching my father make tofu, or bean curd, for the whole community, from beginning to end, with fresh, farm-produced soybeans. First he washed the beans. Then he laid them evenly around the circular wood grooves in the mill. Then the big horse-powered stone wheel would be pulled over the beans for a while. The milled soybeans were washed and filtered into a basin with the leftover rough part saved as food for animals. The balance went through a heating process, then a cooling process. Then the mixture was poured into a square-shaped mold that allowed the water to drain out, thus forming tofu. Somewhere in the process, big heavy stones were put on top of the tofu mixture to compress it, with a piece of cloth as a divider to keep the content clean. The soft, watery tofu, before compressing and molding, is a product itself. Called tofu brain, it is a delicacy served as breakfast, mixed with soy beans boiled with Chinese five spices, and spiced further with oil, vinegar, salt, and a bit of scallion greens. Very nourishing and fragrant.

Tofu by itself is very bland. It gets its life from spices – for example Sichuan-spiced tofu, or from the meaty flavor of a beef stew. If you freeze it in cubes and then use them in a stew, they take on the nice chewy texture of a meat product. Tofu can be used in soups as well. After all the ingredients and flavors are in, just drop the cubed tofu into the soup and bring it to a boil again to cook the tofu.

For vegetarians and vegans, tofu is a very good source of protein. Choose tofu made from non-genetically-modified soybeans whenever possible. Just be sure to read the label. I find the tofu varieties from Chicago's Chinatown are labeled as non-GMO. Here are some quick tofu recipes:

Sichuan spicy tofu (my style):

- One tablespoon coconut oil or any other oil of non-GMO origin
- Two dry red peppers, chopped into fine bits
- Raw ginger, chopped fine, roughly a teaspoon
- Two cloves of garlic, finely chopped
- Sea salt, black and red pepper, and turmeric, to taste
- A tablespoon of rice cooking wine, any cooking wine, or just plain wine
- One package of soft tofu (medium-firm or firm will do if you can't find the soft variety), drained, washed, and cubed, ready to be cooked
- One scallion and a few sprigs of cilantro, finely chopped, for garnishing
- Teaspoon of extra virgin olive oil, for the finishing touch (optional)

- A few drops of toasted sesame oil, for the nutty flavor

Heat up a sauté pan with oil over medium heat. Stir in the raw spices: dry pepper, ginger, and garlic, all together. As soon as the aroma rises, put in the dry powdered spices: sea salt, black and red pepper, and turmeric, then the cooking wine, and then a half cup of water. Bring to a boil. Stir in the cubed tofu and reduce the heat to low to simmer. It will be ready in about ten minutes. Transfer the mixture to a serving plate (I prefer an orange or dark red plate for contrasting color and visual energy). Garnish with the chopped scallion and cilantro. Sprinkle some extra virgin olive oil and the few drops of sesame oil for added nutritional benefit as well as enhanced taste.

Mild flavor tofu: By playing with the red pepper proportion, or with very little or no red hot pepper, you end up with a mild-flavored tofu.

Tofu with black bean sauce: If you are close to Chinatown and can find some fermented black beans, you can simply add a tablespoon of this mixture in with the spices, with or without hot pepper. Everything else can stay the same. Then you have a dish of tofu with black bean sauce.

Homestyle tofu:

- Three tablespoons of coconut oil or any other non-GMO oil with a higher smoke point suitable for pan-frying.
- One package of firm tofu cut into cubes
- A handful of nuts, either almonds, peanuts, or walnuts, chopped fine or ground

- Fresh basil, in small pieces
- Garlic, finely chopped
- Half a white onion, sliced
- One red hot pepper or green hot pepper, sliced (optional if you like it hot)
- Half a cup of white or brown mushrooms, thin sliced
- Half a cup of broccoli, thin sliced
- Salt, red and black pepper, turmeric
- A tablespoon of rice cooking wine, any cooking wine, or just plain wine
- A few drops of sesame oil or olive oil
- Two or three green scallions, sliced or shredded

Heat up a large, flat saucepan. Put in two to three tablespoons of oil. Once heated, put in the tofu cubes, one or two at a time, making sure each has contact with the bottom, until the pan is filled. Keep the heat low to medium to avoiding burning. Adjust the heat based on what's happening in the pan. If there is too much sizzling or smoke, reduce the flame. If there is too little action going on in the pan, turn up the flame a notch. Turn the tofu over with tongs or chopsticks when it is browned on one side. When both sides are browned, take it out into a bowl or a dish for further mixing. Repeat until all the tofu is done.

Rinse out the pan or heat up a clean one with a tablespoon of oil. Stir in the nuts to be roasted, then the fresh basil, garlic, onion, peppers, and mushrooms. Stir a few times. Put in the broccoli and stir a few times. Be gentle and controlled. Spice up the mixture with your salt, pepper, and turmeric. Mix in thoroughly. You can also put in the wine at this time and let it cook a second. Then carefully mix in the browned tofu. Flip the mixture with a big spatula so as not break the tofu. Spice it with your dry spices one more time if needed. Be very cautious with your spices, especially salt. Transfer to a serving plate, garnish with your usual dose of sesame oil or extra virgin olive oil and the scallions. This dish can stand alone or be served with a black/brown/white rice mix or simply a small serving of white rice.

Tofu sautéed with vegetables: This is just an expansion of the last dish, with more of a variety of vegetables of your choice added in. Vegetables that work well with this dish are snow peas, broccoli, bok choy, celery, Chinese cabbage, Chinese broccoli, and peppers. You can replace the basil with raw ginger and turmeric, and everything else can stay the same. It is very delicious and easy to make. You can alter the vegetables and end up with something completely different.

Tofu buns with chives: This recipe does require some time, a spirit of exploration, and some skills in baking. If you are ready and willing, I am behind you with the recipe, my love, and my story. I saw my mom make it a million times when I was growing up. I made it myself in America from pure memory when my belly craved that childhood favorite food and I was missing my mom.

Prepare your dough as you normally would for bread: Use six to eight cups of flour – a mixture of whole wheat flour and white flour. You can add some almond meal flour if you are in the mood, for the extra flavor and the health benefit. Mix one packet of yeast with two cups of very warm water and set aside. Mix the flour with two eggs and a tablespoon of sea salt in a large ceramic bowl. Once thoroughly mixed, slowly pour in some of the yeast and water mixture. Either using your hand or a mixer, constantly mix the dough as the water is being poured in, a bit at a time, until it is absorbed. The dough should not be so soft as to be sticky, yet not so hard to the point of being hard to mix. It should have just the right softness and be easy to knead, feeling soft, bouncy, and smooth.

Knead the dough, constantly, for about ten minutes, either in the bowl or on a clean surface. Then wash the bowl, brush the bottom and sides with oil, and put the dough back in the bowl. Rinse a clean cotton kitchen towel under very warm to almost hot water, squeeze it dry, and spread it over the bowl. Put a plate or plastic wrapping over the bowl to prevent dryness. Let it sit for two hours to rise.

When the dough is almost ready, prepare a pot for steaming. Fill it one inch deep with hot tap water. Oil a steamer tray with coconut or peanut oil or any oil you use in your cooking – organic butter is okay as well – to keep the buns from sticking to the steamer. Now you can make the filling, my mother's traditional recipe:

- One package (1 pound) of firm tofu, cut into small cubes
- A bunch of chives, maybe one pound, picked clean – discard any loose yellow coverings from the stems, washed, and finely cut. The chives can be purchased from Chinatown, but you might be surprised by what you can find at your local market. Last year at my

neighborhood farmer's stand I saw some chives lying there. They were being given out for free, only because the farmer didn't know what to make of them. I was so grateful to have something so special, right there close to home. Chives are not green onions or scallions. They are thinner, with a strong scent, especially after being cut and cooked.

- A chunk of raw ginger, finely chopped
- One tablespoon of coconut oil, melted, or any other oil that is non-GMO with a higher smoke point, such as corn, soybean, peanut, sunflower seed, or pure olive oil
- Pinches of black and red pepper/paprika/cayenne pepper, turmeric
- Sea salt, one teaspoon or to taste

Mix the tofu, chives, ginger, oil, pepper, and turmeric together, and stir well. If all the spices are balanced just right, you should be able to tell by the wonderful aroma that seduces your senses. Wait to add the salt until the wrappers are ready, to prevent a watery condition from developing. To be safe, you can just taste it. (There are several ways to correct an overly salty condition: add in some finely grated carrots; two stir-fried eggs without salt; some other vegetables such as finely chopped Chinese cabbage or regular cabbage; some potato noodles (soft after soaked in water); or a combination of these.)

Now make the dough into wrappers for the filling. This part does take some practice, but you have to start somewhere.

Keep in mind that skill comes with practice, just as with driving. Take half of the dough that is in the bowl and roll it many times over a relatively large, floured cutting board. Once smooth and spongy, roll it lengthwise. Keep rolling it with your palms into a cylinder until it is the width of your wrist. Then use a knife to cut it into chunks, each about one inch thick. (This determines the size of your buns. I personally like big ones with tons of filling.) Spread them one at a time with your rolling stick as you would with any dough wrappers. One hand rolls over the dough while the other holds the dough, moving it counterclockwise to keep it evenly spread. Put them aside, putting enough flour in between to prevent them from sticking to one another – not too much flour, just so it will be easy to seal the edges once the fillings are in – and work on the next until all are done, piled on top of each other.

To make the buns, hold one spread wrapper in one palm and hold a large spoon with your other hand. Scoop up a spoonful of the filling and pile it onto the wrapper, about 60 to 70 percent full. Then tightly seal the dough along the edges with your fingers, or anyway it works for you. I personally like the buns to be very full so that I can enjoy more of the filling, but it's a challenge to seal them properly with the larger amount of filling, due to the somewhat slippery condition resulting from the salt in the mixture making the filling watery; the wrappers can open up in the steaming process. Once a bun is done, put it in the steamer right away, with a small space in between them, until the steamer is filled. You don't want them to be too tight because the dough needs room to rise.

Cover the pot and heat over high heat until steam comes up. Then turn it down to medium heat for about fifteen minutes, and then to low heat for about another ten minutes. Once you turn off the heat, open the lid slowly so the steam escapes gradually, avoiding too much of a contrast between the cold and hot air, affecting the look of the buns. Let them sit for five to ten minutes, or until relatively cooled off. Gently transfer the buns to a serving plate by hand.

You can serve them as is or make some dipping sauce to go with them. The sauce can be a Chinese dumpling sauce I usually make with hot oil over smashed garlic, salt, turmeric, and black and red pepper/cayenne pepper/paprika, mixing well with some rice vinegar and soy sauce, a few drops of sesame oil, and a few bits of cilantro or/and green scallion. Take one bite of the bun, then use your spoon to scoop the sauce up, dripping it into the opening in your bun. Or you can serve the buns with a salad, with the same sauce as a dressing. Or you can sauté some hot green peppers to go with the buns.

Once you master this dish, you can make variations by using chicken, ground beef, or some other vegetables such as hard cabbage or Chinese cabbage. If you have leftover dough, make a loaf of bread with it if you like, simply by spreading the balance of the dough on a floured cutting board in a rectangular shape and rolling it up like long bread loaves you have seen. Tuck the ends under. Place it on an oiled baking pan for about one hour, or until doubled in size. Meanwhile, heat up the oven to 350°. Place a pan of hot water in the bottom of the oven to add some moisture to the heated oven environment. Bake the bread for about twenty minutes, then coat it with either one egg white or some coconut oil and bake it for another twenty minutes, or until done to the degree of brownness you like.

Beef

Steak: Cooking steak is much easier than you might think once you get the hang of it. To begin with, buy clean beef, organic from grass-fed animals that have lived a normal, natural, and happy life. Beef steak can be cooked in a frying pan over medium to high heat. Sprinkle a pinch of black pepper on both sides before the steak goes in the frying pan. Salt when both sides are seared and browned. Salting in the beginning results in a chewy and tough texture. You can sauté some mushrooms, bell peppers, and onions of any color on the side in the same pan. This serves several purposes. First, the tasty moisture content penetrates into the steak, and the beefy taste of the steak flavors the vegetables, making everything taste better. Second, it saves using a second pan. Third, you have a good, delicious, nourishing meal in record time.

Beef Sauté: Sautéing beef is about the same as sautéing vegetables. It's very quick and convenient, cooking within minutes over high heat. A steak cut is ideal and easy to cook. A few ounces serves two or three people. Some vegetables can be added, such as celery, pea pods, Chinese broccoli, broccoli, onions, and bell peppers, mixing in some carrots for visual enticement. Cut the vegetables the same way to create uniformity and visual attractiveness. Use a small cutting board to cut the meat, different from the one you use for vegetables. Then wash it well, with some distilled vinegar, baking soda, or a half slice of lemon. Scrub the board to clean out all the bacteria that could contaminate other food items. Here are a few ideas for beef sauté:

Cumin beef:

- Half pound clean, grass-fed beef, sliced
- Three cloves of garlic, sliced
- Two tablespoons powdered dry cumin
- Sea salt and black pepper to taste
- Two dry hot red peppers, sliced (optional if you like spicy food)
- Two hot green peppers, sliced (optional if you like spicy food)
- A few slices of bell peppers, a mixture of red, green, and yellow is best, but not necessary. The idea is to add in as many goodies as you can without overpowering the flavor or character of the main dish.
- Small onions, sliced

Heat up a saucepan, adding some oil, over medium-high heat. Once the pan gets hot, with the oil melted or hot, stir in the beef. Quickly stir for a few minutes until the beef turns dark. Stir in half of the garlic and the cumin, a little bit of salt, and black pepper. Transfer all to a bowl. Clean the same saucepan, or use a different one, add oil, and heat it up. Put in the balance of the garlic. Let the aroma rise, and then quickly stir in the red and green hot peppers, bell peppers, and onions. Flavor with the rest of the cumin, sea salt, and black pepper, stirring with a wooden spoon or chopsticks a few times. Mix in the cooked beef. Turn off the heat right away to prevent overcooking the beef. Scoop up into a white or cream-colored dish, creating a contrasting energy and vision.

Beef with broccoli:

- Two cloves of garlic, sliced
- A small chunk of ginger, the size of a fingertip, finely chopped
- A small amount of raw turmeric, if you have it; otherwise use dry turmeric powder
- 3 to 4 ounces clean, grass-fed organic beef, thin sliced
- Sea salt, black and red pepper/cayenne pepper/paprika, to taste
- A small onion, cubed
- One medium-sized broccoli crown, broken down into pieces

Heat up a sauté pan or a wok with some oil over medium heat. Stir in half of the garlic, ginger, and raw turmeric. Then put in the beef and turn the heat to high to yield a tender texture. Stir a few times. Spice lightly with sea salt, both peppers, and dry turmeric if you do not have the fresh version. Once the color of the meat changes, scoop it up into a bowl or plate, waiting to be combined with the broccoli. This should be fairly quick, maybe about five minutes.

Clean the same pan, or fetch a clean one. Heat up with some oil over medium heat and put in the rest of the garlic, ginger, and raw turmeric. When the aroma of garlic hits your nose, turn the heat to medium-low, put in the cubed onions, and cook until the onions wilt. Then put in the broccoli. Stir a couple of times. Spice it up with your favorites of sea salt, peppers, and turmeric if you like. Then mix in the cooked beef. Very quickly stir a few times, and then turn off the heat. You can toss in a few drop of sesame oil if you love the nutty flavor as I do.

Beef with peapods or other vegetables: You can add more variety to your beef sauté by adding vegetables such as pea pods, Chinese broccoli, celery, Chinese greens of various kinds, onions, bell peppers of all colors (red, green, purple, yellow), and cauliflower. They also add diversity, raise the nutritional value, and enrich life.

Stewed beef: For tougher cuts of beef, stewing is more appropriate.

- Fresh ginger and garlic, finely chopped
- One pound organic beef cut into bite-sized squares
- Sea salt, pepper, turmeric, and cumin to taste (cumin optional)
- Sesame oil, cilantro, and finely chopped green onions for garnishing.

Heat up a stainless steel medium-sized pot with some oil in the bottom over high heat. Drop the raw ginger and garlic into the sizzling oil, then the square-shaped beef. Quickly sear all sides. Spice with salt, pepper, turmeric, and a pinch of cumin if you like the flavor, which I love with meat products. Then pour a cup of water into the pot, or enough water to cover the food. You can put the covered pot in the oven at 350° for a couple of hours, or you can simply simmer it on the stovetop for about an hour and a half, or until the meat gets tender. Near the end of the cooking process, you can sprinkle some salt into the pot for the flavor to be thoroughly absorbed and mixed in. Garnish with sesame oil, cilantro, and green onions.

Ground beef: You can make burgers, cooking sauce, or your favorite dishes such as lasagna, Chinese dumplings (饺子), meatloaf, meatballs for your sandwiches, soups, or spaghetti sauce. I prefer to spice ground beef with my favorite flavors of sea salt, black and red peppers, turmeric, and cumin. For meatloaf, some cooked rice, finely chopped garlic, basil, and the usual spices mixed in with the beef makes a very nice loaf. When used in other dishes, flavor ground beef in whatever way you like, be it Italian, Chinese, American…. Use your favorite cookbooks. Be bold and creative.

Chicken

Chicken can also be prepared in many different ways. Sauté it as with beef above, matching it up with all varieties of sliced and shredded vegetables. Chicken needs to be thoroughly cooked, yet not overly done.

Pan-fried chicken breasts: Before cooking, marinate with dry spices such as sea salt, peppers, and turmeric by rubbing them thoroughly into the chicken. Then pan-fry each side for about five minutes. If you want them to cook faster, you can slice the chicken breasts thinner before marinating. Once almost cooked, you can turn off the heat and let them sit for a few minutes until thoroughly cooked. You can always cut the chicken open and check for doneness. When it is completely white in color, it is done. If there is a bit of a red color or it looks raw, it needs to be cooked further. You can use it in chicken sandwiches, in a meal as a protein, in salads, or in soups. It can be cooked in the oven as well, marinated with basil, garlic, vinegar, and sea salt to taste.

Baked whole chicken: Marinate the same way, rubbing thoroughly with sea salt, pepper, turmeric, maybe even some cumin. The flavor will penetrate deeper if you let it sit in a bowl in the refrigerator for a while covered tightly with plastic. Better yet, use ceramic bowls that come with covers to save on disposable resources. Ceramic is safer than plastic, and the food somehow comes out tasting better. You can marinade for from one hour to a few days. Not only does it make the food tastier, but it also prevents spoilage, though there is a limit as to how long it can sit. Check for freshness before you cook.

Bake it at 350°F. If you are a busy person, and you have about two-and-a-half hours before you plan to have dinner, preheat your oven to 350° as soon as you get home. Place the marinated chicken in a baking pan. Bake for one hour, and if you happen to have some yams, sweet potatoes, or red potatoes, add them to the same pan and cook another hour. Salad is a perfect complement to a meal like this one. If you are in the mood, you can also have another vegetable such as broccoli, green beans, or kale.

Baked chicken legs, drumsticks, and quarters: Chicken legs need less time to cook than a whole chicken, so prepare as above and check often for doneness, making sure there is no blood or redness showing in the juice inside of the chicken.

Chicken soup: Chicken soup is especially nice in the winter, to build, nourish, and boost your immunity. It is actually quite easy to make as long as you have some time on your hands for the traditional method. If you don't have time to babysit the soup, invest in a slow cooker. Then you can go about your eight-hour day, and when you get back it is hot, steamy, delicious, and ready. Here is how to get the soup going:

- Small to medium chicken
- Raw ginger, chopped into small chunks
- Three cloves of garlic
- Raw turmeric, finely chopped (or the dry powder form)
- One dry hot red pepper, if you like some extra zest
- Sea salt and black pepper to taste towards the end (For a slow cooker, you can add these at the very beginning or at the very end. Keep in mind that spices added at the beginning penetrate into the chicken, becoming part of it.)
- Two green scallions, finely sliced for garnishing, or cilantro, or both

Fill a large stainless steel pot with water to about 75 percent full. Put the chicken into the pot, completely immersed in water. Bring to a boil and use a ladle to skim any bubbles off the top. Turn the heat to the minimum. Put in the ginger, garlic, turmeric, and dry hot pepper and slowly cook for a couple of hours. After one hour, season with salt and black pepper so the flavor can be thoroughly absorbed. Once the chicken gets tender and breaks up easily when being poked with a fork, turn off the stove. Serve the broth with the finely chopped scallion and/or cilantro in a bowl as soup, with or without the meat. The rest can be refrigerated and heated on an as-needed basis. You can also use the broth as a soup base for other soups such as noodle soup, vegetable soup, and rice soup, or whatever your heart desires or the availability of ingredients dictates.

Eggs

Eggs can be scrambled, boiled plain or with five spices (the way the Chinese do it), deviled, or sautéed with vegetables. To make with vegetables, flavor the raw eggs with a bit of sea salt, a pinch of black and cayenne peppers, or paprika and turmeric. Scramble the eggs by pouring them into heated oil in a flat pan. Flip a couple of times, using a flat flipper. Once the watery eggs transform into soft, solid eggs, scoop them up into a plate or a bowl. The cooked eggs can then be mixed with vegetables sautéed as above in the section on vegetables. I normally don't add milk or water to the raw eggs for eggs with vegetables as I would for scrambled eggs served as breakfast.

Fish

Fish can be grilled, pan-fried, steamed, or poached. For salmon, a little sea salt and black pepper sprinkled on both sides will do very nicely. For poaching, simply put the cleaned fish with a bit of water in a frying pan. Turn on the heat to medium. Place a few slices of raw ginger, garlic, and green onions alongside in the water so that the flavoring from the herbs can penetrate the fish, enhancing the flavor and adding nutritional benefits. Fish is very easy to cook through. About five minutes will do. If it is very thick, both sides might require three to five minutes each. Be sure to check with a fork. It should be juicy, oily, tender, and easy to break off.

Grains

Grains are a staple in many cultures. They can be cooked with liquid as porridge or without excess water the way rice is served in a restaurant.

Porridge: I grew up with porridges for breakfast almost every day, from split, rough corn porridge to finer corn porridge and millet porridge, and further diversified with combinations of different beans such as mung beans, red beans, soybeans, etc. After years of staying away from them, I have been incorporating porridge into my breakfast again. It is very simple to prepare. Rinse some grains in the pot you will be using for your porridge, and then drain them. With the grains in the pot, fill it up with water to about half full – usually about a half cup of water to one cup of grains, depending on the thickness of the porridge desired. Put the pot on the stove over high heat. Bring to a boil. Turn the heat to the minimum, covering the pot half way. Let it slowly simmer, the emerging fragrances permeating the air. Stir with a ladle from time to time to prevent sticking. You can always precook the porridge the previous night and simply heat it up the next day. Here is a special recipe I love:

Rejuvenating black rice porridge:

- Small handful of black rice
- Small handful of sticky rice (a variety of white rice with a stickier nature; can be replaced with brown rice, regular rice, or pink rice)
- Small handful of dry black beans
- Small handful of dry red beans (optional)

- Small handful of dry pearl barley
- About ten pieces of dried lily bulbs (an herbal ingredient loaded with nutritional and medicinal value; can be purchased at some oriental stores)
- Small handful of peanuts or walnuts
- Five to seven dates, pitted and hand broken into loose pieces (optional)
- Half handful of black sesame seeds
- Sugar made from plum tree sugar in solid form, or any other form of organic sugar, loose or in solid or crystal form (in solid chunks)
- One small-sized banana, sliced (optional)

The night before, rinse everything except the black sesame seeds, sugar, and banana. You can rinse out the black sesame seeds if you have a very fine strainer; otherwise use them as is without rinsing to prevent the seeds being washed down the drain. Put all the rinsed ingredients in a medium-sized pot. Fill it with water to about two-thirds full. Now put in the black sesame seeds and turn the heat on high. Bring the mixture to a boil, then turn the heat to low and simmer for about ten minutes. Turn off the heat. Cover the pot well and let it sit on the stovetop overnight. The next morning, add a teaspoon of sugar and the slices of banana before cooking if you crave a bit more sweetness. If you are an early riser, you can always cook the porridge after you get up in the morning, getting it to the point of simmering before you go about your morning routine of self-love and self-care, but be sure to soak the beans overnight. The porridge will need to cook for about two hours.

There are many multigrain porridge mixes in the food stores in Chinatown. The most popular one has eight grains and is called porridge of eight treasures. You can always add dates, cubed sweet potatoes, apples, dried grapes, bananas, dried haw flakes (haw is known for digestion), and some healthy form of sugar into the mix for a bit of sweetness.

A word of caution: It is okay to start most grains in cold water, except buckwheat and oats. They get mushy, with no texture. Add these to boiling water instead.

Solid grains (including rice): Measure about two cups of grain and rinse. Add the grain and two cups of water to a pot and bring to a boil over medium-high heat. Then turn the heat to low. Simmer about thirty minutes without stirring. This retains an undisturbed look; once stirred it has the look of thick porridge, especially Chinese rice.

You can invest in a pressure cooker, which will stop automatically once the thickness and pressure come to the right point. You can also use an electric rice cooker, which also stops automatically. Have it sit for about five to ten minutes after it is cooked on the warm setting after it automatically turns to warm or stops. This will give the grain the opportunity to settle in, with consistency and thickness.

Fried rice or grains: With the busy lifestyles so many of us lead, it is very convenient to have a pot of rice or grains of various kinds already cooked and kept in the refrigerator for later use. It can be revitalized and turned into something delicious and nutritious in record time. Here is my quick recipe for two or three servings to get you started:

- Tablespoon of oil
- One clove of garlic, finely chopped (optional)
- A bit of raw ginger, finely chopped (optional)
- A small piece of turmeric, finely chopped (or dry powdered turmeric)
- One small onion, any color will do, chopped fine
- Three white button mushrooms, diced (optional)
- Half cup of broccoli, sliced
- One small carrot prepared in small cubes
- Pinch of salt and pepper (black, red, or cayenne pepper or paprika) to taste
- Pinch of cumin (optional)
- One cup of cooked rice or grains
- One egg, scrambled
- One scallion, finely chopped, for garnishing (optional)
- A bit of cilantro, finely chopped, for garnishing (optional)
- A few drops of sesame oil, for finishing flavoring (optional)

Heat up a wok with oil. Once the oil is melted or heated, put in all the raw spices (garlic, ginger and turmeric). Quickly stir a few times. Then put in the onion and stir again. Then the mushrooms, and stir a few times until the mushrooms and onion get tender, wilted, and soft, with a delicious onion aroma in the air. Add the broccoli and carrot. Move it quickly a few times. Spice the mixture with salt, pepper, and cumin, mixing in thoroughly. Then mix in the rice and egg. Flip with a wooden flipper to be sure the rice and other ingredients are thoroughly mixed. Taste it to see if more salt is needed. Garnish with scallion, cilantro, and sesame oil. Shrimp, chicken, or beef can be added to make it a complete meal. Meat products should be cooked first and set aside for combining. You can always add cubed peppers of any variety as well.

Legumes and Beans

This is another good food group for the living microbes in your gut. For easy digestion, it is a good idea to soak legumes and beans for a day or two, or for at least one hour, before cooking. Some of the smaller beans do not require presoaking. You can leave them plain or salt them towards the end of the cooking time, giving them enough time to be cooked thoroughly without the salt prohibiting them from being properly cooked. You can also spice them with cumin to reap the benefits of stimulation and aid in proper digestion by reducing the gassy condition and the feeling of stomach bloating, which usually accompanies bean consumption. A pinch of turmeric can be added as well, for the added benefit of cooling and reduction of an inflammatory condition. Some herbs such as cilantro and finely chopped onion can be cooked with the beans, too.

Bring the beans to a boil in a large pot of water about 75% full, and then simmer over low heat for one to five hours, depending on the size and nature of the beans. For example, mung beans cook quickly, while lima beans and other hardy beans take much longer. Once cooked, beans can be served either by themselves as protein or along with a vegetable and maybe a small amount of meat. They can be mixed in with salad, in wraps with meat and vegetables, in soups, or in any other creation of your own.

Laomian noodles: I am often asked how to cook this Chinese dish. If you are skilled working with dough and able to make noodles from scratch, do just that. To prepare the dough for the noodles, mix one cup of flour with water. Gradually stir in the flour, with one hand holding the water cup while the other hand mixes the flour. You can always use a mixer for this task. Be sure to be slow and thorough, so as to not add too much water. You can spend a full ten minutes playing with the dough, like the way a child plays with Play-Doh. Once smooth and bouncy, cover it and let it sit.

Now prepare your vegetables, meat, and/or eggs to have with your laomian noodles. Here are the ingredients:

- Two tablespoons of coconut oil or any other good cooking oil, one for cooking the meat and egg and one for sautéing the vegetables
- Small chunk of raw ginger, finely chopped
- Two large cloves of garlic, thinly sliced
- Small piece of raw turmeric, the size of a lima bean, finely chopped
- An ounce of meat (pork, chicken, beef, shrimp, etc.), shredded in the same shape as the noodles you see in restaurants for uniformity and visual appeal. You can actually use all of these meats, like the house dish in

many restaurants, or just one; less quantity of each if you choose to have them all

- Salt, pepper, both black and red/paprika/cayenne pepper
- One egg
- Half of a small onion, sliced
- Three to five white or brown mushrooms, sliced
- A stalk of celery, thinly sliced
- One small to medium carrot, shredded
- Half cup of cabbage, thinly sliced
- Tablespoon of soy sauce
- Tablespoon of rice wine vinegar, balsamic vinegar, or any other cooking vinegar
- One green scallion, thinly diced, for garnishing
- A drop or two of sesame oil, for the finishing touch

Heat up a saucepan or a wok with a tablespoon of oil. Once heated, quickly put in some of the raw spices: the ginger, garlic, and turmeric. Flip very quickly. Then toss in the meat. Stir a few times. Flavor lightly with sea salt and peppers. Stir a few more times and transfer it to a bowl. It should look cooked at this time. Shrimp should look pink; chicken and pork, white; and beef dark red. Set aside for final combining. If you choose to use all the meats, they are better cooked separately so that none of them is either undercooked or overcooked.

Scramble the egg and set it aside to be combined in the end, when the noodles are ready.

In a clean, large wok or saucepan, heat up a tablespoon of oil. Once heated (when you drop some vegetables in the oil, they sizzle right away), put in the balance of all the raw spices and quickly stir a couple of times. Put in the vegetables, onions, and mushrooms first, and move with your wooden spoon a few times. Then put in all the remaining vegetables, one by one or all together if they are on the same cutting board. Let it sizzle a few minutes, flipping a few times. Then turn off the heat and let them sit to be combined with the noodles when they are ready.

Now take out the dough you have sitting in a bowl, sprinkle some flour on the surface of a large cutting board or other flat surface to prevent the dough from sticking, and lay it out on the board. Start kneading the dough with your two hands, back and forth, until it is smooth, round, and bouncy. Then push it outwards and forwards with your palms. Once the spread becomes too big for your palms, start to roll it with a rolling stick. Keep sprinkling dry flour onto the dough and the surface as needed. You can roll the dough up around the stick, push it over the board from one end to the other, then open it up and start over again. Keep repeating the process until the spread is thin enough for noodles. You can spread it until paper thin, or maybe a bit thicker, depending on your liking.

When the dough is thin enough, you can fold it over to a length that you can cut with your cutting knife. Add enough flour so the layers don't stick together. Cut along the folded dough to make the noodles, the same way you shred your vegetables. Pick up the noodles with your hands, loosen the noodle strands from the folds, and gently lay them down flat on an empty part of the board you are working on. Make sure they are loose and not sticking together.

Fill a medium to large-sized pot about 65% full with cold water and bring it to a boil over high heat. Gently put the noodles into the water, one handful at a time, keeping them from sticking together. Stir with a wooden utensil. Once the water returns to a boil, the noodles should be ready if they are very thin. If they are thicker, pour a half cup of cold water in the pot and bring it back to boiling. Taste a noodle for doneness. If done, turn off the stove and rinse the noodles under cold running water to inhibit further cooking. This will prevent the noodles becoming too soft without any chewy texture left. Carefully eliminate all the excess water from the noodles by using a strainer of some sort. Sprinkle some oil on the noodles to keep them loose, ready for the final combination.

Now mix in the noodles with the cooked vegetables in the same large saucepan the vegetables are in, and add the prepared scrambled eggs and meat. Heat up the pan and stir gently from the bottom up with a large flipper. Salt and pepper to taste. If you like a bit of soy sauce or vinegar, you can add this as well, no more than a tablespoon each to avoid overpowering. Then scoop it up into serving plates, garnishing with scallions and sesame oil.

You can always buy some ready-made oriental noodles, dry or wet, from a market nearby, to be boiled at home. Then combine with your vegetables and meat. Spaghetti noodles work fine if you cannot find the oriental variety. The dried version normally takes longer to cook than the wet version. Al dente is the ideal state for the noodles, soft to the lips and chewy to the bite.

4. Assemble Your Three Meals

The Chinese saying "Eat like an emperor for breakfast, king for lunch, and beggar for supper" pretty much sums up how we should be treating our meals. Chinese wellness promotion and Ayurveda tradition support this philosophy.

Breakfast should be substantial and nourishing after more than twelve hours of fasting. I normally break the fast with a bowl of my black rice porridge or any other version of whole grain/bean/nut porridge, along with an egg, pan fried with or without vegetables or boiled and deviled. Sometimes I have just my home-style omelet – egg batter over sautéed vegetables cut into small cubes. Ingredients range from some or all of the following: ginger, garlic, mushroom, onion, tomato, broccoli, basil, and leafy greens.

A combination of fruits, oatmeal, and juice works, too. Watch out for too much sugar intake. Fresh fruit juice intake normally should not exceed one glass. If you have pre-diabetes or acute diabetes, it's wise to stay away from fruits, especially for breakfast. Fruits are not free as far as the sugar content is concerned. Blueberries are one of the best, with their very low sugar content. Check with your health-care provider for more information about whether or not you should eat fruits.

Regular bread, a bagel, or an English muffin is okay, though whole grain versions are always better than those made with refined flour. You should have something to go with it, such as an egg or some clean meat, to slow down the absorption of the carbohydrate load. If you feel tired and sleepy after eating bread, a bagel, or a muffin, ease off and have this every few days. Again, bread is not a good breakfast choice for people who are prone to diabetes or have it already.

Smoothies and juice blends of various vegetables and fruits are good, too, especially for summer days. These are normally just a side dish for me because I move a lot, and I love my meals to be warm, solid, and delicious.

Cereal with milk works too, as long as it is a healthy kind. Go by the ingredient list, not the health claims from the company.

Lunch should be substantial as well, large enough and sustaining enough to tide you over until suppertime. It can be a combination of all the food groups, heavy on low-starch plant-based foods such as a variety of vegetables, cooked in any form; a serving of protein, either a meat product or plant-based, such as beans; served with a small portion of grains. The less processed, the better.

The sautéed dishes above with a combination of meat, tofu, and vegetables are very handy, with a small serving of brown rice, white rice, or wild rice, or a combination. Recently I have been combining brown rice with regular rice in my rice cooking – two parts brown rice, one part white rice – healthy yet tasty.

The laomian dish by itself is sufficient for lunch, offering a bit of everything.

A salad with the oven-roasted chicken recipe above is good, too. The salad can consist of ingredients such as nuts, fruits, leafy vegetables, onions, slices of tomatoes, cucumbers, avocados, or a combination of them all.

Sandwiches of various kinds work, too – fish, chicken, beef, or egg salad, along with loads of vegetables. It is always good to have soup to go with a cold meal, adding warmth and satiety. The chicken soup recipe above, made ahead and ready in your refrigerator, is very handy.

A homemade noodle soup is great for lunch, too. Sometimes I sauté some base vegetables as in the above recipes – the ones that are good in soups such as mushrooms, tomatoes, onions, carrots, or a stalk of celery with garlic, ginger, or basil – then fill the pan with water, bring them to a boil, add noodles of any variety, the healthier the better, boil until the noodles are cooked to the right tenderness, and turn off the stove. Finish up with some sesame oil, vinegar, soy sauce, and finely chopped green scallion or cilantro. If you have leafy greens or Chinese greens, you can always boil some with the noodles and serve with the meal. Make sure the portion of noodles is moderate. Vegetables, especially the leafy greens, can be as much as you want. If you like some meat in it, add some during the sautéing, putting the meat in before the vegetables. Some basic flavoring can be added while sautéing, with adjustment in the end. Sometimes I cook the noodles separately. Once they are drained, I spice them up with some crushed garlic, extra virgin olive oil, a little bit of vinegar, soy sauce, a pinch of salt, and some finely chopped scallion, and serve them with a dish of vegetables of any variety.

The challenge is when you work outside of the home. This is normally when I eat at a restaurant, making the best choices under the circumstances. If you work at an office, you can always take a dish you prepared earlier and warm it up there. It's ideal if your workplace has a toaster oven. Ceramic containers are the best to hold your lunch.

Supper should be supplemental, just as the name suggests. It can be anything, just less than at breakfast and lunch. If you don't feel hungry, you can skip the meal. Ayurveda even suggests that.

Chapter Ten

Detoxification

Detox is quite the buzzword these days. Even if you don't pay attention to media and online advertisements, you hear the word somewhere. It is a good concept, and serves us as the beings we are if it is approached the right way and with the right intention.

Most detoxification programs focus on diet, from the extreme of drinking just water to mild ones that include light meals. But it is so much deeper than that, focusing on the truth of who we are as spiritual beings living human experiences.

Emotional Detox

When I see someone walking around looking angry, tired, and depressed, I feel this surge of compassion, finding myself responding quietly, "Poor soul! What is it that is triggering you to behave this way?" At one IIN yearly conference, Joshua Rosenthal, founder and educator of the school, demonstrated how much emotional burden we had all been carrying, beating us down and making us tired, angry, and depressed. He put one small bag on one shoulder, then another bigger one, then another even bigger one, then a large-sized travel bag on the other shoulder, and a carry-on bag around his neck. At last he picked up a chair and held it over his shoulder. We carry so much emotional baggage – the make-believe stories, the hurt feelings, the broken marriage, the relationship long overdue, the unwanted child, the not-good-enough, or the not-know-enough. By the end of the day, this emotional bondage drains everyone, leaving us depressed, despaired, barely keeping up, and not in any position to embrace life as a whole person. Like many of my colleagues and IIN community friends, I was in a bucket of tears. I simply sat there, allowing the tears to roll freely down my cheeks, literally feeling lighter.

We come to our physical bodies with souls that have chosen to experience certain things in life. Naturally we are bound to have many of the ups and downs, lows and highs of life, with the emotional impressions of it all imprinted on our subconsciouses. To fully live the lives we are born to live, it is essential to go through life burden-free and tap into the unlimited potential that is ours to have, in whatever ways we choose to be.

These emotional burdens stem from the belief systems, conditioning, expectations, and perceptions we experience from the day we are yelled at or looked at in a certain way to this moment. The deep reason we experience these burdens is the separation from source, from one another, from self. The societies we live in often encourage us, especially men, to keep our emotions to ourselves. It is considered a flaw in character to show emotions. Many of our parents hide their emotions. We learn from an early age to guard against them, not allowing anyone in on our emotional secrets.

Many of us silently suffer from emotion-induced toxins – physically, emotionally, mentally, and spiritually. For the longest time I fought battles instead of savoring life and living true to myself. I suffered needlessly. The emotional baggage I carried could very well have been the bodily weight that manifested on my physical body, let alone the heaviness that constantly sat on my heart, rendering me depressed and miserable.

When you start to realize there is something much bigger and deeper than the surface reality you are experiencing, you naturally gravitate your way home – home to love, to oneness, to unity, and to bliss. To be there, to feel at home where you belong, you naturally start going through the process of digging through layers of conditioning – the misperceptions, the insecurities, the blaming, the anger. Once there, you shine your light, like the sun; that light, that brilliance, that magnificence, that essence of love has been in you all along, ready to come through as soon as there was enough clearance, just like the sun shining its light once the clouds are out of the way.

Once you start this detoxifying healing process, you experience patches of your light, your wisdom, and your greatness coming through. You might find yourself in awe of your power, marveling at the brilliance of the universe, grateful you are part of the magic cosmic whole. You might choose to witness more of it firsthand by constantly observing and healing, learning to let go of the made-up stories that did not exist to begin with, and fully owning up to your life, your happiness, and your destiny. Blame no one, judge no one, expect nothing from anyone, detach from being a slave to social norms, and start living from your heart and soul, with that inner gut intuition as your guide. Apply that same principle in loving yourself up in every way possible. Simply observe, reflect, learn, and apply.

On days when you feel low, being weighed down by the dense energy around you, bear in mind that your light is there, waiting for the dense fog to clear away, just like the sun is always there above the clouds. You can simply hunker down and walk through the clouds to reconnect with your light and shine. Here are some of the reflections and coaching suggestions I offer my coaching clients and the practical applications I live by:

- **Peel the onion, feel the emotions, and then watch them melt away, layer after layer after layer, until you are nothing but light and love.** Emotional intelligence is taught in colleges now and has been embraced by many. It is essential for our soul's further evolution. Basically understand that your emotions are here to teach you. Direct them in ways they can serve you as the person you are instead of giving them free reign in running your life. Every time you catch yourself feeling sorry for yourself, or feel toxic emotions such as anger, disappointment, overwhelm, hatred, jealousy, resentment, stress, or depression building up, first allow yourself to feel it. Let it brew in you; feel its force running through you. Observe how it is developing and rising, and how it affects your body. Where is it in your body that you feel it? How does your body react to it? How old is that part of you that feels that emotion? Then go to that space and comfort that hurt child from where you are now by physically hugging the place in your body where you feel the emotion. Then observe this display by stepping back as if you are watching a movie. By doing so, you are honoring your feelings while detaching yourself from them, by being the silent witness you truly are. You will soon discover that you are so much more than your emotions.

Afterward, look at it from the perspective of the person or situation that triggered the emotional trauma. You might find yourself thinking, *Maybe there is another way to look at this. Just maybe he or she could be right or the situation is not as bad as I am making it out to be.* You might have just gotten yourself into a corner. The majority of the toxicity might be gone at this point. Then you can look at it again through the neutral lens of a third party. You might even wonder why you got yourself all worked up to begin with. Chances are some of the toxic emotions are still there, recurring time after time.

Talk it over with a trusted friend or a trained professional who does not exercise judgment. Sometimes I am prepared to go over the benefits of vegetables and how to cook them, but my client wants to talk about cooped-up emotions, troubled relationships, or the challenges of building up a heart-centered, passion-driven business. I just sit back, be present, hold the space, and allow my client to lead and talk things through. Never underestimate the healing power of having someone listen to your troubled emotions, especially a trained professional, which is healing in and of itself.

My coaching client Liz certainly enjoys the benefit of having a coach guiding her through this process. Here is an email from her sharing her sentiment and her emotional growth:

Hi Sue,

Thank you so much, I loved our session last night. I can't quite believe how content I feel so much more of the time. I am so grateful to have met you and to have been on this journey with you.

I was just looking over my notes for last time, and I saw there was a note to ponder on what I can be or do so that my mum can be what she is supposed to be and honor my space. I realized that what you said about just being myself and being steady is already helping her – and me – and, in fact, me having strong boundaries teaches her to build her own and to trust me, as well as herself. I think this might just be the biggest gift I can give her, and I am so happy to have realized this. Thank you.

I love the thought of embracing and not running away from the things and people I am afraid of; I feel nervous, but there would be such freedom in not having to run away. I feel like the knowledge and awareness are becoming one. I will keep practicing all of our work. Thank you so much, lots of love and hugs, xxx

Often it is necessary to ask for help. For example, if you can't convince your whole being to happily carry on the task of doing dishes and all the household chores on top of carrying the responsibility and honor of putting food on the table and a roof over your head, then obviously your family needs to get involved for a solution. Explain to your loved ones how you feel, ask everyone to pitch in to help you be the healthier version of you, and be there for them, physically, mentally, emotionally, and spiritually.

Even after I had looked within, deeply immersed in my essence, and talked my emotions over in different coaching settings, I still felt resentment for carrying so much on my shoulders. After much commotion and emotional eruptions, I involved my family, explaining that I should feel happy that I was fortunate and healthy enough to do what I did, but that many times I didn't; that I felt taken for granted; that the fact that I was willing to do all these things shouldn't be taken so lightly and everyone should actively participate. Gradually some of the cooking, cleaning, and merchandise preparation has been taken off my plate. I have even found my laundry done and the folded clothes on the ironing board. The cat litter boxes have been changed more often, and their eating area seems to be much neater and tidier as well. It feels really good to walk into a house that is somewhat clean and in semi-order. It is not only the cleanliness, tidiness, and somewhat clutter-free space I love to see, but with this improvement I find my resentment, anger, and frustration further melting away.

To further eliminate the detrimental, unhealthy impact this toxic emotion has on you, you can practice some sort of ritual such as writing the whole experience down, then burning it, envisioning the toxic emotion gone with the smoke while you mentally let go of its hold on you, starting fresh.

It is imperative to face your emotions head on instead of avoiding them by sweeping them under the carpet. Sooner or later, if not already, they show up in your physical being. Or you might experience the feeling of being worn-out and fatigued that no amount of sleep can adequately address. Or you might simply explode, yelling and screaming. There are times you might be severely depleted and exhausted just from carrying these emotions with you. By addressing these toxic emotions promptly, you will not only avoid adding more to the layers and layers of built-up toxic emotions already there, but also facilitate the healing process by peeling them off once they surface. This enables your body to function more optimally, allows your heart to open up more for more loving and uplifting vibrations, and frees up

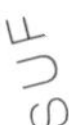

more space for the things of your deepest
flow in.

Every emotion is stored in your cells as memory. Therefore, give your emotions your attention, love, and space. Honor them. Respect them. They will melt away, out of your system, a little at a time, a layer at a time, until they are gone. Once you are on this healing path, it is part of an ongoing process, releasing you from the built-up burdens, enabling you to move forward light-hearted, with a lighter load and razor-sharp focus, to live the way you are meant to live – whatever way that is.

- **Stay away from the very toxic people** in your life whom you can't help, especially when you are fresh in your new light and the dense, toxic emotions and energies might pull you down, leaving you feeling fatigued and depressed. Give yourself enough time and space for that energy to ground and entrench. Find the company of those who radiate light and love. Read books that inspire and resonate with you deeply. In the meantime, keep all your self-love and self-care routines going strong and steady to keep building up strong muscle and resilience in its totality – body, mind, heart, and soul.

- **Look for the lessons**. Every person in your life serves as a mirror, reflecting part of you. Instead of getting upset with what they say or do, ponder and reflect the messages for you. Those of us who are on our unique paths often hear people telling us it is too late for us, how idealistic we are, how we can't possibly sustain doing what we love, how we need to have a normal job. Could that be simply mirroring back to us some part of us where we feel insecure? Let that be the guide for continuous inner polishing and reconnecting.

- **It is not always about you.** Chances are it is them, not you, when people make remarks, judgments, and behave towards you in a certain way. People around you might be emotionally burdened, with tons of baggage and garbage. It could be a bad day for your boss when he criticizes you. The clerk who was rude to you might have had very little sleep that night due to the many hours he worked to support him and his family. Your partner who was impatient with you could be feeling that way with himself or herself, and you happened to become the target of that frustration. Don't always take it on you.

- **Focus on you.** Leave others alone to find their own way out of the matrix home. All too often our anger comes from loved ones living a certain way. They might be eating toxic food, going to bed late, staying on the couch watching TV for hours on end, drinking excessively, complaining about everything, or blaming everyone for their misery. You want to help them. You know the stuff is bad for them. You hate the way they live; the way they think. But they can't see things the way you see them. Leave them alone for the time being. Instead, use all that energy on yourself, applying self-care and self-love in all areas of life. Eat right, treat yourself right. Do yoga stretches, meditate, and think supporting thoughts. Never put yourself down. Don't be modest by playing small. Live up to your dreams instead of scaling them down. Focus on being that person you want to see more of in this world. After a while, you become more vibrant. More glow appears on your face. You smile often, you laugh more, you seem happy… you have created a bubble in you and around you. People in your life can't help but notice that happy radiance in you, through you, around you, in your aura. Some might respond by following your lead. Some might shy away from it. Some might want to have what you have. Now it is time for you to show them how it is done. Chances are the right audience will listen now because they see the truth of you through your living example.

Eat to Cleanse

Your body is amazingly intelligent with millions of years of evolution. Trillions of cells are working in harmony, communicating, defending, responding, and watching out for one another, even sacrificing themselves to keep the host body at optional functioning. What you put in your body at what time each day and at what intervals plays a big role in keeping that marvelous living organism functioning smoothly and seamlessly, or having it work against you by impairing your body's innate function of keeping your body performing at optimum.

We are exposed to all sorts of toxins, from the food we eat to the air we breathe, the chemicals spread on lawns, and the by-products our bodies produce just to go about our daily living. In this sense we are truly in it together, with one person's or one industry's behavior affecting everyone else. It is a chain reaction, one thing leads to the next, another leads to another. It is imperative to break the pattern, beginning with ourselves. The most logical place is what we put into our mouths, day in and day out. Here are the things you can do to keep your body relatively clean and burden-free, giving your liver more power to filter things through:

- **Start eating clean foods**; this was addressed in the food-shopping and food-choice section above.

- **Eat three meals daily**, gradually phasing out the snacks in between meals. This allows your body time to digest your food properly. It also offers your body a whole night to cleanse the whole system. Start the day with a hearty breakfast to break the overnight fast. Enjoy a lunch good enough to last you until a light dinner, at least two hours before bedtime to digest most of the load for better sleep and cleansing.

- **Try a light or liquid diet.** If you are a busy person, and you are looking for some cleansing, you can just eat lighter meals, consisting mostly of vegetables. If you have the flexibility to stay at home and do this at your own pace, you can experiment with a liquid diet. Only consume foods such as soups. Make your soup and remove the solid foods such as vegetables and meats after the soup is done cooking. This will give your digestive system a proper chance to relax while still taking in enough nutrients for sustenance.

Some people cleanse by only drinking water for a weekend, spending the whole time lying down, drinking water, and going to the bathroom. Some who tried this told me they felt weak during the weekend and renewed come Monday morning after it was over. Meals can be gradually resumed with soups first, then solids, easing into normal meals towards the end of the week.

If you are feeling good and have a good appetite, vibrant energy, and vitality – if you are at your optimal health and weight with no apparent digestive issues – you can simply keep your normal meal routine and fast for twelve hours each day, from about 6:00pm to about 6:00am (sundown to sunrise) if you work a traditional daytime schedule, give or take a few hours' deviation. This is how our world's natural civilization functioned and evolved. Once farming began, with steady food supplies, our ancestors lived this way. There are populations that are still living in harmony with nature, using nature as a guide to align their life's daily cycle. In my hometown, most people are still doing the same, with no outwardly apparent physical health problems.

There is a Chinese detox recipe that is promoted and practiced by some of the Daoism followers. I once read on WeChat about a doctor using Chinese cabbage to treat his many heavily constipated patients and getting very good results. A Dao monk later confirmed that cabbage had been used over the years to clean out a blocked digestive system. It pulls toxins out of the liver, helps bulk up stools, and removes toxins, along with other undigested matter, through bowel removal. The ideal duration for this detox is three days, consuming only boiled Chinese cabbage (白菜) leaves whenever you are hungry. Then drink the cabbage juice on the third day. As elimination begins, dark feces come first, then yellow ones. Very colorful ones containing toxins come last. It is even better if you can do it for one week each month. According to the Dao monk, it is best done over a weekend.

I experimented with it a few times, thinking that it was only Chinese cabbage, a wholesome vegetable, so it wouldn't cause any harm. The first day it was okay, but I had to have other foods with it because it was too intense for me. I felt nauseated. My understanding is that the scraping effect in the digestive system is too strong for me, probably because my diet was already relatively clean and my digestion was in good working order; there was probably not too much there to get rid of. My Chinese doctor friend verified this after a visual and pulse session. I had mentioned this cleansing method to him. He remarked that all the leafy vegetables would offer similar benefits. I intend to get at it sometime again when I have a block of a few days available. In the meantime, I frequently add Chinese cabbage to my vegetable intake.

Sweat It Out

Your skin is the biggest surface area for removing toxins from your body. It can be sweating from hot weather, a workout, mowing the lawn, gardening, or doing yard work – just about anything that makes you sweat, which of course includes a hot sauna or steam room. If the temperature is tolerable, use nature as air conditioning instead of sitting in a cold, air-conditioned car or living in an ice-cold house. Keep the windows of your car and your house open, and sweat while you move about. Have a nice shower or bath at the end of the day to wash the toxins off your skin. If you sweat profoundly, wash it off right away, leaving no opportunity for the toxins to be reabsorbed. Sweating also opens your pores and keeps your system breathing. Drink plenty of water to replenish lost water content.

Create a Cleaner Environment

- **Find creative ways to keep your lawn beautiful naturally, without using chemicals to kill the weeds and dandelions.** I often wonder about the waste and the biologically harmful environmental effect we are unconsciously having on ourselves and future generations. It harms our living companions such as our dogs, cats, and birds, and the worms and microbes that live in the soil. If you should ever think of planting a garden and having your very own vegetables and fruits, using chemicals should be the last thing you would want to do. The chemicals reduce the microbe diversity in the soil and result in fewer nutrients in foods. This, in turn, gives you less building power. You would also be missing out on feeding the trillions of microbes that live in your gut helping you digest food properly and keeping your immunity stronger and your brain sharper and clearer. To me, a natural-looking lawn with wild-looking flowers is a sight to behold. It is much safer for my daughter and our house cats and anyone who passes by. It is healthier for the atmosphere we are all dependent upon for vital life force as well.

Somehow we have gotten it backward. We try to kill something hardy, local, and beneficial and replace it with something that takes much effort to maintain and too much water to nurture.

Maybe what needs to change is not the weeds in the lawn, but the way we view things. View it from the perspective of natural evolution, the law of survival. What happens if we eat something so hardy and hard to kill? Does that make us stronger, more resilient? Those studying *food energetics* are saying this. We as eaters take on the quality of our food, whatever that might be.

- **In your home, use safer alternatives** in cleaning your dishes, floors, and clothing. Even if you wear plastic gloves when you use chemical-laden dish detergent while washing your dishes, you inhale much of the toxins floating in the air. So the best thing is to use something safer. Hot water alone is sufficient for cleaning lightly used dishes. I use a chunk of lemon, vinegar, or baking soda to clean the rest. They all cleanse. They smell clean and are highly hygienic. The same can be used for mopping floors, using a solution of hot water and vinegar or baking soda, or simply a mop and hot water.

- **For your body, facial, and hair products, the same mindful approach applies**. The guiding principle is anything not safe to put in your mouth should not be used on your face or skin. I alternate between cooking oil, coconut oil, aloe, and sometimes some very common and inexpensive alternatives such as Ponds or Oil of Olay everyday facial cream and Jergens Ultra Healing moisturizer. Last winter I purchased some Arbonne botanically-based facial products. They are working well so far. I alternate these choices to stretch my dollars. Someone from a company selling healthy facial products told me that the most important factor for facial products is the balance of acid and alkaline ingredients. After using their product for just a day or two, red spots appeared on my cheeks. I am not saying their product is not good or they were lying to me, but your skin composition is as unique as your whole person, your digestive tract, your immunity, and the way your body responds to stress. Some in the health industry say your skin functions as a huge absorbing surface. It soaks up everything it comes in contact with and carries it into the bloodstream without the benefit of the liver as a filter. In a way, it is worse than ingesting through the mouth to the digestive tract, the liver, the bloodstream, and all parts of the body, with the remains as feces to be removed.

stew, they take on the nice chewy texture of a meat product. Tofu can be used in soups as well. After all the ingredients and flavors are in, just drop the cubed tofu into the soup and bring it to a boil again to cook the tofu.

For vegetarians and vegans, tofu is a very good source of protein. Choose tofu made from non-genetically-modified soybeans whenever possible. Just be sure to read the label. I find the tofu varieties from Chicago's Chinatown are labeled as non-GMO. Here are some quick tofu recipes:

Sichuan spicy tofu (my style):

- One tablespoon coconut oil or any other oil of non-GMO origin
- Two dry red peppers, chopped into fine bits
- Raw ginger, chopped fine, roughly a teaspoon
- Two cloves of garlic, finely chopped
- Sea salt, black and red pepper, and turmeric, to taste
- A tablespoon of rice cooking wine, any cooking wine, or just plain wine
- One package of soft tofu (medium-firm or firm will do if you can't find the soft variety), drained, washed, and cubed, ready to be cooked
- One scallion and a few sprigs of cilantro, finely chopped, for garnishing
- Teaspoon of extra virgin olive oil, for the finishing touch (optional)

increase the other flavoring ingredients by about one spoonful if you like more flavor.

You can fish out just enough for one meal at a time – a condiment-sized serving to go along with your main dishes. It takes some trial and error to get just the right combination. It helps to start small, maybe one-half to one pound of vegetables, until you get the hang of it. It benefits the bugs in your gut, and therefore your health. It is good for your wallet, too. Have fun experimenting.

Chinese Tofu: I grew up watching my father make tofu, or bean curd, for the whole community, from beginning to end, with fresh, farm-produced soybeans. First he washed the beans. Then he laid them evenly around the circular wood grooves in the mill. Then the big horse-powered stone wheel would be pulled over the beans for a while. The milled soybeans were washed and filtered into a basin with the leftover rough part saved as food for animals. The balance went through a heating process, then a cooling process. Then the mixture was poured into a square-shaped mold that allowed the water to drain out, thus forming tofu. Somewhere in the process, big heavy stones were put on top of the tofu mixture to compress it, with a piece of cloth as a divider to keep the content clean. The soft, watery tofu, before compressing and molding, is a product itself. Called tofu brain, it is a delicacy served as breakfast, mixed with soy beans boiled with Chinese five spices, and spiced further with oil, vinegar, salt, and a bit of scallion greens. Very nourishing and fragrant.

Tofu by itself is very bland. It gets its life from spices – for example Sichuan-spiced tofu, or from the meaty flavor of a beef stew. If you freeze it in cubes and then use them in a

Chapter Eleven

Feed Your Cravings

Embrace Your Appetite

Cravings are driven by unmet needs that derive from hunger and desire, two ends of the same spectrum that have been driving the biophysical body in its evolution. Hunger is on the low end and desire on the high end; one feeds the other, being equally important. Hunger and desire are the driving forces that propel you to choose one food over the other. The physiological drive is very intuitive and instinctive, and it is a natural demonstration of your life force. True desire reflects your deepest yearnings. It is not simply the desire for your basic needs, but the desire that is behind your entire existence and is your appetite for life.

Psychologist Abraham Maslow's *Hierarchy of Needs* details human needs from basic to higher growth needs, ranging from the most basic biological, physiological needs to the highest of transcendence needs, and all other needs in between – safety, love and belongingness, achievement, meaning of life, beauty, and harmony. Humans have been driven by unmet needs from survival to sex, love, life purpose, peace, beauty, and giving. Often we end up looking for satisfaction through foods.

Your relationship with food is a reflection of your relationship with your life. Your every emotion, impulse, and action innately seeks out the imbalances that exist in your system – mind, body, heart, and soul. Many of the unmet needs in the form of cravings and strong desires are looking for ways to be compensated, maybe through binge eating or sexual promiscuity, to make up for a lack of satisfaction; unfulfilled desires, wishes, and dreams; or a lack of real power within. Satisfying a craving is not as simple as just giving your body the food and keeping it full for a little while. It has a much deeper dimension, tied to all areas of life. When you reach for that donut, is it really your hunger that drives you or is it something totally different? Could it derive from a habit of eating donuts for breakfast with the memory in your cells habitually reacting a certain way? Or is it that you are missing something sensual in your relationship, that passion and intimate closeness? Or is it something missing from your life you can't quite put your finger on – you know it is there because it drives you restless, but on the surface everything seems to be just fine with a good family, a beautiful home, and a good business or secure job? Or is it something so important, so vivid, that the fiber in your very being craves it to make you the person you want to be in this life?

You come to this lifetime with a soul wanting to live certain experiences through your physical body. This creates a certain set of wants, needs, and desires needing to be fulfilled. Any overlooked need or want creates an imbalance in your life that can show up as a food craving. It is a symptom of dissatisfaction with life or body image, or simply being out of place. Sometimes it drives you to do certain things to stay occupied and busy, avoiding understanding or facing the true issues in life. That is why the diets out there usually don't work. As much as they focus on choosing the right food with the right calories, they solely depend on will power, going against the strong innate desire. If you can stay on such a diet for a lifetime and be successful, by all means go for it. But if you are not enjoying the whole process of living, what is the point? Aren't you missing the point of coming into this life to live your magnificence, to stretch out of your comfort zone, to experience exhilaration, joy, and bliss?

If any one area in your life is out of sync or out of yin-yang balance (阴阳平衡) according to the Chinese yin-yang philosophy, it will show up somewhere. It might be in your eating, or in doing something you wouldn't otherwise be doing to compensate for the feeling of lack and insecurity or to avoid the unshakable sense of being a failure.

The answer is simple: Feed your craving, whatever it is. Be it food, relationship, too much uptime with a lack of downtime, too much doing with a lack of being, too much spiritual with a lack of physical intimacy and closeness with another being, or vice versa. So many of us attempt to suppress our healthy appetites for food and for life. We get bombarded by the tips out there about how to curb our appetites to lose weight. How is that helping in the long run? It is not even natural. A healthy appetite is a sign of robust health and a love of life, where food is the most basic element, spiritual enlightenment the ultimate aspect, and all the other aspects of life falling somewhere in between. Once the belly is full, our attention is driven to other needs and desires. It could be for proper living conditions, companionship, love, or the highest form of self-realization: simply being in love in oneness.

The key is to be intimate enough with yourself to know exactly what your appetite is for, then feed it accordingly. Avoid feeding a much deeper craving with food as a substitute, which can never address the real issue. We are supposed to experience life to the fullest. Good appetite means your body is healthy and craves good fuels to sustain, continue, emerge with new life, uncover new dimensions, reveal new meanings, and discover new insights. It is this driving universal life force that is expressing itself through you in your appetite for food and life, with food and eating playing a big part in sustaining your physical life. It is essential to find the right things that quench that hunger, thirst, and desire for life.

With a constant here-and-now awareness, observe your cravings and understand them for what they are. Find ways to feed them to honor yourself as the eater and as the being you are – body, mind, heart, and soul. If you truly want that food, go ahead, give your body what it wants and desires. If it is that fat donut, by all means have it. Savor every bite with leisure, with appreciation, and with gratitude. Allow the sensation of each bite to spread through your five senses, washing over you. Be fully present with that moment of sensual satisfaction. Never regret what you have just done. Be grateful you have the wisdom to honor your cravings instead of fighting them.

There is a very interesting theory that thoughts of food can make a person fat. The reasoning is food anticipation starts with the brain, which triggers the secretion of the hormone insulin to digest loads of sugary carbohydrate, real or imagined. Unused insulin is stored as fat deposited in tissues. This is called *cephalic-phase insulin response*. So it is better to eat it and get it over with. Then at least your insulin has something to work on instead of being secreted for nothing but adding to fat storage, inhibiting muscle growth, and gaining weight without even ingesting any calories.

Reflect on these theories about cravings and see if you can find something a bit healthier to satisfy yours. Maybe a nice honey-coated apple or dark-chocolate-coated strawberries. Maybe a bar loaded with nuts, seeds, and other goodies wrapped in dark chocolate. Maybe something as simple as a bite of fruit or carrot, or just a sip of water. Perhaps it could be something other than food, such as a chat with a dear friend, a good book, a nice walk. Maybe it is investing some effort in improving the relationship you are avoiding facing. Or something spiritual like looking within, connecting more deeply with yourself, or figuring out the purpose of being in this lifetime.

Overindulging and suppressing are the two extremes. The sensible thing is to indulge with awareness, understanding it for what it is. Tantra, a branch of Buddhism, says, "The lower needs are not to be denied; they are to be transformed into the higher." This is not to say go ahead and forget about everything else and give in to your bodily needs and impulses; it says to listen to your body, honor your body, and respect its innate wisdom and knowing. Indulge so you can go beyond the bodily needs to the knowing that you alone are the source of your bliss, originating from that source of everlasting cosmic orgasm.

It is here where the enlightened come down to mundane life, living drunk in happiness, always laughing. They carry with them a radiance and vibration we know are not of this world. Denying or suppressing that is like blocking our life energy and spark. It is a delicate dance. The goal is the beautiful middle, neither overindulging nor oversuppressing. Constant observing in awareness, and gut intuition, will guide you through. The lower needs are the basic needs that drive us as human beings: food, safety, and sexual desire. Allow all your needs and desires to be your guide in feeding your cravings and, in the process, learning the truth of that which you are.

Chapter Twelve

Build, Modify, and Maintain a Supporting Daily Routine

All the things we have covered so far – mindset, lifestyle, and foods – mean nothing if you do not incorporate them into your life. In the end, it is what you do on a daily basis, day in and day out, year in and year out, for the balance of your life, that defines the quality of your life, for better or for worse. Once healthy practices become part of your life, living is as easy and effortless as putting one foot in front of the other, the way driving becomes second nature and breathing is your involuntary life support. There is no need for struggling, especially if this comes from your source, your center, something you have consciously chosen because you know its building quality in your bones. It becomes an integral part of you, embodying you. In essence, it is all these things. As you may realize already, you can't really go wrong with a healthier lifestyle. Find that spark and fire – that which compels you to get up in the morning, dream dreams, and crave things – that makes you hungry with a strong, healthy appetite for food, for life, for love, for compassion, for anything in life.

It is said a lifestyle habit takes about twenty-one days to develop, about six months to become established, and just one day to be interrupted. Once you set the habit, following it is a breeze. All you do is just do it, be with yourself, and show up for yourself, without analyzing, without thinking it over, and without making excuses. Your brain and your body have memory cells everywhere. This explains why even though you don't think you know how to do a certain thing, your body sometimes does it automatically. New cells grow as well, with new ways of thinking and new patterns of doing things in the new daily habits. Your brain literally forms new grooves and maps out new patterns of thinking, feeling, responding, and acting.

Over time, you fulfill your deepest desires, living from that center which is the spark of the universal life force. Don't force yourself into something you hate, creating stress and defeating the purpose of the habit-building practice. Identify things that benefit you and support you as the real person you are to build youth and vitality. Once you feel the uplifting sensation coming from feeling naturally high, you will be motivated to do more.

Assemble Your Daily Routine

It's very important to factor in everything about you in creating your daily routine. Your new routine should be a way of life you can live by for the balance of your life. It is essential to hold that vision of where you want to see yourself in one year, five years, or ten years, or the legacy you want to leave behind. This might be the very reason to stay on track with a sustaining, supporting lifestyle and daily routine.

Let's suppose you yearn to be a writer, downloading all that is within you, through you. Then obviously you would want to have some structure for getting the message out day by day. Let's suppose you want to feel young, look young, and be young; then a youthful, robust mentality and way of life need to be part of your daily routine. You are not going to be naturally slim and have a healthy body weight as a by-product of living if all you do is sit on the couch watching TV all day long, stuffing calorie-laden, colorful, artificial stuff mindlessly into your mouth. What you put in is what comes out – the beautiful law of energy exchange. The minute you start incorporating daily baby-step routines into your life, you start living your dream. Persistence makes that vision into a reality.

Incorporate into your lifestyle the things you do on a daily basis, such as your three meals, the way you digest your experiences and emotions, and the baby-step actions you take towards your life purpose. It can be your sleep quality, time, and duration. Your bodily movements to build strong muscles and bones and increase heart capacity are part of routine-building as well.

You can start with just one thing or two things. As I normally recommend to my coaching clients, you should decide on a maximum of three things to add in for two weeks, then add three more after the two-week period. Habits to add could be a few minutes of meditation, a few yoga stretches, maybe going out running until you sweat, working out at a gym, and switching to sipping hot water instead of morning coffee first thing after you get up.

If you are a busy person, you can simply add some leafy greens to your meals without changing anything else to start out. Add an after-lunch or after-dinner walk to your routine. Or a power nap after a big lunch, to give your body some time to properly digest the food while most of your blood is directed to the digestive tract area.

Play with your kids more. Maybe it's that vegetable garden you want to get going, moving your body while producing something organic and benefiting your belly from your own labor of love. Maybe it's the flight of stairs you climb instead of using the elevator to and from your office. Park your car farther away from the store when shopping on your way home from work. Maybe it is the lead-generating marketing funnel you will focus on after you have gained clarity and youthful vitality.

The beauty is, you can choose to change anything important to you. You can look, learn, observe, test-run, and pick and choose what feels right to you, and then experiment with it to see how it works for you. Simply stick to it for a while, for the habit to sink in, and see its beneficial effect on you as a whole person, both emotionally and physically. As long as your schedule permits, keep at it.

Modify Your Routine as Life Happens

Modify your routine from time to time to accommodate your growing changes. Life is dynamic. The only unchanging fact is constant change. Things happen; so will your daily routines. As long you have the awareness that routine habit is what makes or breaks whatever you want in life, you will be able to assemble all the pieces into the new puzzle at any given time.

You might want to add some walks in the outdoors with the change of seasons – snowy, cold winter turns into warm, breezy spring, when the outdoors comes to life: buds form, grass turns greener, bushes shoot up. You might choose to change your job, your schedule, or some routine in your household. Maybe your kids start pitching in with the laundry, opening up possibilities for something you want to do for a while but you haven't been doing due to your long list of to-dos.

You can modify your daily habits as often as is needed. Choose just one to start with to set things in motion. Be disciplined enough to stay with a good, workable routine, yet flexible enough to make changes when changes are necessary. There is no need to get stressed over establishing a new routine. The whole idea of having a sustaining routine is that you can live a healthy, stress-free life by simply following the flow you have created in the first place, and then modifying as life happens. It's your life, so let your routine work for you to build the quality of life you dream of living.

Be mindful of the following in your routine-building, modifying, and maintaining process; some of these points have been covered in the corresponding chapters, summarized here to facilitate your routine-building process:

- Bodily movement in the form of functional or non-functional exercises in the early part of the day sets your metabolism for the day, even though it is very beneficial to stay active throughout the day. The traditional wellness philosophy recommends staying active in the early morning when your body is mostly alert.

- Move your body for the benefit of overall well-being in building muscle mass, bone density, and lung and heart capacity, increasing your body's innate ability to build quality blood. You will have a boosted immunity to fend off alien invaders and activate a deep, consistent repairing and restoring mechanism.

- Let your body be your guide as to when and how much you move your body. It should be enough to invigorate, yet not so much as to deplete and exhaust you. Those with blood type O are born with more durability for exercising, therefore it makes sense for them to engage in vigorous aerobic exercise. Those with blood type A are easily tired out, so practice gentle exercises such as qigong, yoga, and golf.

- You can always add calorie-light, nutrient-dense foods such as a fresh salad loaded with leafy greens to your meals regardless of what you are eating and how busy you are. In the long run it will make a big difference in your health in balancing your homeostasis, embracing your food cravings, and keeping your body healthy and fit.

- Never underestimate the accumulated effects of daily habits. I remember hearing someone say that we often overestimate what we can do in days and underestimate what can be done in years. This struck me to my core. It's so true. Just observe the successful people you admire and the ordinary people in your life. Are they that much different? Do the successful ones know more or are smarter or luckier than the less fortunate ones? You know the answer to that – it's a big NO. There is not much difference at all. It is all in our daily habits.

- Fully appreciate nature and its wisdom, honor your body as part of a divine whole, and deeply respect and follow nature's ebb and flow, cycles, and principles as the Vedic premise "As in the macrocosm, so in the microcosm" tells us. Always consult nature in everything you do in the here-and-now awareness. That includes eating what is supplied by mother earth in its most basic forms; listening to your body's innate intelligence – its needs, wants, cravings, and impulses – the spark; stopping eating when your body says "full"; going to sleep shortly after night falls, getting up and moving when it's bright and sunny outside; putting more clothing on when it's cold instead of turning the heat up to 80°; and turning off both heating and cooling when it's nice and comfortable outside.

- Be aware not to stress and crowd your mind while you are in your daily habit of building health, youth, and vitality. Simply allow the new habit directed by the new grooves in your cells to naturally take over. During self-care, give it 100 percent of your attention. Be fully present with it – body, mind, heart, and soul. Regardless of what it is, make it an end unto itself.

When you become aware of your mind racing ahead, overthinking the day ahead, making plans, or worrying about a certain aspect of it, stop that by taking a few deep breaths, bringing your attention back to your breath, and getting centered and grounded again.

- Be patient in building your lifelong lifestyle habit. There is no need to rush it in one day just to forget about it the next. Take baby steps. Add one to a maximum of three new things at any given time, gradually easing them into your routine until the habits stick.

- An accountability partner in the form of a friend, spouse, or coach is very helpful in establishing and maintaining a supporting routine. Being part of a group-coaching program is a very good way to approach routine building as well. That way you not only benefit from having a guide on the side, but also a group of peers sharing their journeys and experiences, holding space and encouraging one another.

- Keep at it, even at times when you don't feel like it. The act of carrying on with your habit might be the very thing to get you in the groove, kick-start your day, and get the flow going. Just show up and follow the flow with ease and effortless grace. No struggles, no worries, no decisions, no controls. Just let go, with the flow.

- Get back to it as quickly as you can, if you get off. Life happens. When I travel, sometimes it is just not possible to keep my daily routine. I still maintain some semblance of it whenever possible, understanding whatever little I do will keep my overall health at its best. One day does not make a differencc; it is countless of these one days for the balance of your life that make the difference. Don't feel bad or guilty if you get off. Just get back at it again.

Robust, vital health is not only a divine right; it is a divine responsibility. Be the health you want to see. Change the world, starting with you! Let today be the day you start raising your vibration for yourself, for your loved ones, for the world we are all sharing. Not only will you feel young and vibrant again, but you will also lift up those around you with your youthful vitality and happy vibration. This is the best gift you can ever give yourself and the universe as a co-creator – to be the healthiest version of you!

Thank You

Thank you from the depth of my depthless soul and the bottom of my bottomless heart for supporting me by reading about the lifestyle that has transformed my life and countless others. Sharing my message inspired me to get up every day with love in my heart, passion in my being, and fire in my existence, tirelessly rippling the healing effect. If you find the message igniting the fire inside of you, inspiring you to be who are you meant to be, please leave a review on Amazon. Much love and gratitude.

If you are interested in finding out how to work with me closely, please go to my website at www.youngmindyoungbody.com to fill out a health history form and I will get in touch with you for a fifty-minute complimentary strategy session – a gift to you for loving yourself enough to invest in yourself the time you so deserve.

Feel free to sign up for my free newsletter at www.sueziang.com. You will receive a free gift as soon as you submit the form, and weekly or biweekly tips for living your most vibrant life.

With love and blessings,
sue

Sue Ziang, H.C.
Board Certified Holistic Health Practitioner
YOUNG MIND YOUNG BODY Health Coach
Certified Medical/Primordial Qigong Teacher
www.sueziang.com
www.youngmindyoungbody.com

Endnotes

Kaul, Prashant, et al. "Meditation acutely improves psychomotor vigilance, and may decrease sleep need." Behavioral and Brain Functions 6.1 (2010): 1.

Adams, Bruce. Prophet or Madman. Trinus, 2005. Print.

Davidson, Richard J. The Emotional Life of Your Brain: How Its Unique Patterns Affect the Way You Think, Feel, and Live—and How You Can Change Them. Plume, 2012. Print.

Hanson, Rick. Buddha's Brain: The Practical Neuroscience of Happiness, Love and Wisdom. New Harbinger Publications, 2009. Print.

Wu, Qingzhong. The User's Manual for Human Body. Da Guan, 2005. Print.

Singh, Simran. Conversations with the Universe. SelectBooks, 2013. Print.

Epstein, Paul. Happiness through Meditation. Peter Pauper Press, Inc., 2011. Print.

Benson, Herbert. The Relation Response. HarperTouch, 2000. Print.

Batmanghelidj, Fereydoon. Water Cures: Drugs Kill: How Water Cured Incurable Diseases. First ed. Global Health Solutions, 2003. Print.

Pollan, Michael. In Defense of Food: An Eater's Manifesto. Penguin, 2009. Print.

D'Adamo, Peter J. Eat Right for Your Type: The Individualized Diet Solution to Staying Healthy, Living Longer & Achieving Your Ideal Weight. Berkley, 1996. Print.

Spirituality for Dummies, Sharon Janis, Wiley Publishing Inc., 2008.

References and Resources

Books

There are so many books that have impacted me deeply and shed insight on some of the ideas expressed in this book. I have only selected a few here for your easy review.

Benson, Herbert and Klipper, Miriam. The Relaxation Response. HarperCollins Publishers, 1975, 2000. Print.

Braverman, Eric R. Younger You: Unlock the Hidden Power of Your Brain to Look and Feel 15 Years Younger. McGraw Hill, 2007. Print.

Chopra, Deepak M.D. Ageless Body Timeless Mind: The Quantum Alternative to Growing Old. Harmony Books, New York, 1993. Print.

Chopra, Deepak M.D. and Simon, David M.D. Grow Younger Live Longer: Ten Steps to Reverse Aging. Harmony Books, New York, 2001. Print.

Chopra, Deepak. Perfect Health: The Complete Mind/Body Guide. Harmony Books, 1991. Print.

D'Adamo, Peter J. Eat Right for Your Type: The Individualized Diet Solution to Staying Healthy, Living Longer & Achieving Your Ideal Weight. Berkley, 1996. Print.

David, Marc. Nourishing Wisdom: A Mind-Body Approach to Nutrition and Well-Being. Bell Tower/New York, 1991. Print.

Douillard, John. The 3-Season Diet: Eat the Way Nature Intended: Lose Weight, Beat Food Cravings, and Get Fit. Three Rivers Press, 2000. Print.

Gagne, Steve. Food Energetics: The Spiritual, Emotional, and Nutritional Power of What We Eat. Healing Art Press, Rochester, 2008. Print.

Graham, Linda. Bouncing Back: Rewiring Your Brain for Maximum Resilience and Well-Being. New World Library, 2013. Print.

Green, Bob. 20 Years Younger: Look Younger, Feel Younger, Be Younger! Little, Brown and Company, 2011. Print.

Ornish, Dean. The Spectrum: A Scientifically Proven Program to Feel Better, Live Longer, Lose Weight, and Gain Health. Ballantine Books, 2007. Print.

Osho. The Spiritual Path: Buddha Zen Tao Tantra. Ixos Press Limited, an imprint of The Ivy Press, 2007. Print.

Pollen, Michael. In Defense of Food: An Eater's Manifesto. Penguin Books, 2009. Print.

Roizen, Michael F. and Oz, Mehmet C. You Staying Young: The Owner's Manual for Extending Your Warranty. Free Press, 2007.

Singh, Simran. Conversations with the Universe. SelectBooks, 2013. Print.

Smith, Jeffrey M. Seeds of Deception: Exposing Industry and Government Lies about the Safety of the Genetically Engineered Foods You Are Eating. Yes!Books, 2003. Print.

Tolle, Eckhart. The Power of Now: A Guide to Spiritual Enlightenment. Namaste Publishing and New World Library, Novato, California, 1999. Print.

Vallyon, Imre. The New Planetary Reality: The Coming Avatara & The Nine Paths to Enlightenment. Sounding-Light Publishing Ltd., June 2012. Print.

Weil, Andrew. Healthy Aging: A Lifelong Guide to Your Well-Being. Alfred A. Knopf, 2005. Print.

Online Resources

Some of the online resources have been included here for you to dig deeper should you choose to. One way or another, they have enriched my life and the book.

http://www.alongerhealthylife.com/about-us/, secrets to a longer and healthier life, Diane Haworth and Michael Varbaek, longevity researchers, Centenarians walk their way through a longer healthy life, Posted on July 1, 2012, by Diane Haworth

http://www.transparencymarketresearch.com/weight-management-market.html, Weight Management Market by Services, Supplements, Diet, Equipment and Devices: Global Analysis and Forecast (2007 – 2015)

http://www.nbcnews.com/id/36716808/ns/health-diet_and_nutrition/t/when-you-lose-weight-gain-it-all-back/#.VQ9E9DIo7cs, Women's Health, by Gretchen Voss, updated 6/6/2010 12:50:30 PM ET

http://www.goodreads.com/quotes/144557-resentment-is-like-drinking-poison-and-then-hoping-it-will

http://medical-dictionary.thefreedictionary.com/stress+response, Stress Response

http://www.stress-management-for-peak-performance.com/stress-response.html, Stress Less Living, Stress Response

http://www.mayoclinic.org/healthy-living/stress-management/in-depth/stress/art-20046037, Mayo Clinic, Healthy Lifestyle, Stress Management, Chronic stress puts your health at risk; Chronic stress can wreak havoc on your mind and body. Take steps to control your stress, by Mayo Clinic Staff, July 11th, 2013

http://www.allheartattack.com/statistics.php, Heart Attack statistics, All about heart attack statistics worldwide and in the United States

http://psychology.about.com/od/statesofconsciousness/p/TheoriesofSleep.htm

http://www.naturalnews.com/012352.html, The hidden dangers of caffeine: How coffee causes exhaustion, fatigue and addiction, Tuesday, October 11, 2005, by Dani Veracity. Learn more: http://www.naturalnews.com/012352_caffeine_coffee.html#ixzz3brg2iIvU

http://www.differencebetween.net/science/health/difference-between-adrenaline-and-cortisol/, Difference Between Adrenaline and Cortisol, Adrenaline Vs Cortisol

http://scienceblogs.com/neurophilosophy/2008/08/27/wilder-penfield-neural-cartographer/, Wilder Penfield Neural Cartographer, Posted by Mo on August 27, 2008

http://www.danielgoleman.info/, Emotional intelligence, social intelligence, ecological intelligence

https://chopracentermeditation.com/experience, Chopra Center Meditation

http://www.biomedcentral.com/content/pdf/1744-9081-6-47.pdf, Meditation acutely improves psychomotor

http://www.nmr.mgh.harvard.edu/~lazar/Articles/Lazar_Neuroreport_00.pdf, Functional brain mapping of the relaxation response & meditation

http://www.relaxationresponse.org/publications/index.htm, Herbert Benson. Publications and Scientific Research on the Relaxation Response and Meditation. Harvard Medical School. Dr. Benson has been a pioneer in studying the physiological changes during meditation techniques since 1968 as a professor at Harvard helping them become acceptable topics of study.

https://www.upaya.org/uploads/pdfs/MeditationandtelomereEpelANYAS2009.pdf, Can Meditation Slow Rate of Cellular Aging? Cognitive Stress, Mindfulness, and Telomeres. Elissa Epel,a, Jennifer Daubenmier,b, Judith Tedlie Moskowitz,b, Susan Folkman,b, and Elizabeth Blackburn

http://www.bloomberg.com/news/articles/2013-11-22/harvard-yoga-scientists-find-proof-of-meditation-benefit, Harvard Yoga Scientists Find Proof of Meditation Benefit

http://tcmbasics.com/basics_5elements.htm, Traditional Chinese Medicine Basics, The Five Elements Theory https://theory.yinyanghouse.com/theory/chinese/five_element_nutrition_theory, Yin Yang House, TCM Nutrition – Five Element Theory

http://www.greekmedicine.net/

http://www.newscientist.com/special/gaia, James Lovelock and the Gaia hypothesis

http://www.jameslovelock.org/ James Lovelock

http://www.ancient.eu/Greek_Medicine/

http://www.livestrong.com/article/155363-sleep-muscle-recovery/, Sleep & Muscle Recovery, Last Updated: Dec 18, 2013 | By Becky Miller

http://psychology.about.com/od/statesofconsciousness/p/TheoriesofSleep.htm. Theories of Sleep, By Kendra Cherry – Psychology Expert

http://www.whfoods.com/genpage.php?tname=foodspice&dbid=66, Whole wheat (Redirected from Whole wheat flour)

http://www.wisegeek.org/what-is-wheat-germ.htm, What Is Wheat Germ?

http://www.dummies.com/how-to/content/the-human-digestion-process.html, The Human Digestion Process (or, What Happens after You Eat Food), By Carol Ann Rinzler and Ken DeVault from Heartburn and Reflux For Dummies

http://www.culturesforhealth.com/lacto-fermented-daikon-radish-garlic-recipe, Lacto-fermented Daikon Radish with Garlic http://www.mommypotamus.com/fermented-radishes-a-recipe-for-thyroid-healing/, Fermented Garlicky Radishes

http://gnowfglins.com/2011/05/17/naturally-pickled-lacto-fermented-radishes/, Naturally Pickled Radishes — Lacto-Fermented

http://gnowfglins.com/2009/06/03/lacto-fermented-naturally-pickled-turnips-and-beets/, Lacto-Fermented (Naturally Pickled) Turnips and Beets

http://www.motherearthliving.com/cooking-methods/the-surprising-health-benefits-of-fermented-foods.aspx, Fermented Vegetables. Make Your Own Tasty, Digestion-Enhancing Blends at Home, By Michael O'Brien, September/October 2003.

http://www.thenourishinggourmet.com/2009/04/benefitsoflacto-fermentation.html, Benefits of Lacto-Fermentation, April 20, 2009 by Kimi Harris

http://www.marksdailyapple.com/fermented-foods-health/#axzz3YLt9vJ6v, the Definitive Guide to Fermented Foods, Primal Living in the Modern World, Mark Sisson

http://www.rasmussen.edu/degrees/health-sciences/blog/healthy-lifestyle-quotes-to-inspire-you/, 21 Healthy Lifestyle Quotes to Inspire You, by Jennifer Pfeffer on 7/19/2012

http://www.thetotalwellnessdoc.com/benefits-exercise/;

http://www.progressivehealth.com/natural-diuretics.htm, Natural Diuretics That Reduce Swelling, Brad Chase

http://www.oprah.com/health/The-Allium-Family-Dr-Perricones-No-2-Superfood, Dr. Perricone's No. 2

Superfood: The Allium Family. Read more: http://www.oprah.com/health/The-Allium-Family-Dr-Perricones-No-2-Superfood#ixzz3Qp1GU6fJ

http://www.nutrition-and-you.com/vegetable-nutrition.html

http://www.truthaboutabs.com/glycemic-index-carbohydrates.html

http://www.mayoclinic.org/healthy-living/weight-loss/expert-answers/water-retention/faq-20058063

http://www.kitchendaily.com/read/best-oils-baking

http://www.potatogoodness.com/all-about-potatoes/potato-fun-facts-history/, Potato History and Fun Facts

http://healthyeating.sfgate.com/three-functions-fat-body-3402.html, Three Functions of Fat in the Body, by Melodie Anne Coffman, Demand Media

http://www.oliveoilsource.com/page/chemical-characteristics, Olive Chemistry

http://www.healingdaily.com/detoxification-diet/olive-oil.htm, Olive Oil's health benefits

http://www.facethefactsusa.org/facts/the-sweet-life-and-what-it-costs-us

http://authoritynutrition.com/top-10-evidence-based-health-benefits-of-coconut-oil/, 10 Proven Health Benefits of Coconut Oil (No. 3 is Best) by Kris Gunnars

http://www.naturalnews.com/029202_olive_oil_smoke_point.html, Know the Smoke Point for Macadamia, Walnut, Coconut and Olive Oil, Thursday, July 15, 2010 by Fleur

Hupston, Tags: olive oil, smoke point, health news

http://www.goodeatsfanpage.com/CollectedInfo/OilSmokePoints.htm, Cooking Oil Smoke Points

http://www.antioxidants-for-health-and-longevity.com/cumin-health-benefits.html

http://www.globalhealingcenter.com/natural-health/benefits-of-cayenne-pepper/, 17 Health Benefits of Cayenne Pepper. Published on June 21, 2010, Last Updated on May 5th, 2014

http://www.whfoods.com/genpage.php?tname=foodspice&dbid=74, the World's Healthiest Foods, Black Pepper

http://www.organicauthority.com/health/11-health-benefits-of-cinnamon.html, November 29, 2010, by Andrea Manitsas, Energetic Health

http://www.livestrong.com/article/347582-what-are-the-health-benefits-of-curry-powder/ What Are the Health Benefits of Curry Powder? Last Updated: Feb 18, 2014 | By Karen Curinga

http://healthyeating.sfgate.com/healthy-benefits-fresh-herbs-7871.html. Healthy Benefits of Fresh Herbs, by Jan Sheehan, Demand Media

http://www.drfuhrman.com/default.aspx, Dr. Fuhrman, Smart Nutrition, Superior Health

http://www.foxnews.com/health/2012/04/04/healing-power-mushrooms/, The healing power of mushrooms, by Chris Kilham, published April 04, 2012, FoxNews.com

http://www.healingmushrooms.com/, Healing Mushrooms and Medicinal Mushrooms

http://www.empowher.com/cancer/content/healing-properties-mushrooms?page=0,2, Healing Properties of Mushrooms

http://www.healthandwealthtopic.com/2007/09/health-benefits-of-hot-peppers.html,

http://chriskresser.com/diabesity-the-1-cause-of-death-and-disease, Diabesity: the #1 cause of death and disease?, by Chris Kresser

http://www.marksdailyapple.com/top-10-favorite-herbs-and-spices/#axzz3TcsE7k00, Top Ten Favorite Herbs and Spices

http://www.ewg.org/foodnews/

http://www.diabetes.org/diabetes-basics/statistics/, Statistics about Diabetes Data from the National Diabetes Statistics Report, 2014 (released June 10, 2014)

http://www.simplypsychology.org/maslow.html, Maslow's Hierarchy of Needs, by Saul McLeod, twitter icon published 2007, updated 2014

http://wholegrainscouncil.org/node/5903/print, Whole Grains Council, Growing Quinoa

About the Author

Sue Ziang, H.C., passionately supports stressed-out, worn-out entrepreneurs who are sick of being tired and ready to claim their lost youth and vitality and prosper in all areas of life. She came onto the path of healing after she reversed her own "whole nine yards" of the modern-day American epidemic, including weight challenge, diabesety, brain fog, severe depression, anger, extreme fatigue, and feeling lost without meaning and purpose in life.

Sue experienced firsthand the transformational power of supporting mindset, lifestyle, and food choices in everyday mundane living. She witnessed numerous lives transformed in her community, including those of her own coaching clients, by applying the transformational approach she and her community have been living by.

Sue is an AADP Board Certified Holistic Health Practitioner and an Institute for Integrative Nutrition trained health coach. She is an enthusiastic student of Chinese medicine and is currently apprenticing with Dr. and Professor Huang from Shanghai Medical School in Chinese medicine (Dr. Huang used to take on PhD medical students when he was actively teaching), Chinese herbal healing, Chinese acupuncture, and Chinese medical massage therapy. She is currently certified to teach primordial qigong and is training to receiving certification in several more qigong forms.

She brought with her to America a natural-born, healthy lifestyle, a true understanding of the healing power of living in sync with nature and one's natural environment, a deeply-rooted passion, and a conscious knowing in embracing cooking and food as a way of sensual living as well as nourishment, disease prevention, and robust health-building. Sue touches lives with her high vibration of love as a being living in alignment with her core essence. Her deep knowing of one's purpose in life has enabled her to dramatically lessen, erase, and eliminate mind-induced stress and its detrimental effect on her own well-being in a world bombarded with a stress-induced epidemic.

In conjunction with her cross-cultural background, her MBA training, years of running her own business, and teaching experiences, Sue has committed the fourth chapter of her life to rippling her healing effect to others while she lives as a live model of her life's calling.

Sue is currently open to a limited number of highly qualified coaching clients in her six-month signature coaching program. Fill out and submit a Health Form following the link at http://youngmindyoungbody.liveeditaurora.com/forms, if you feel you are an entrepreneur by heart and want so much more out of life, yet have no strength to go after your dream due to the burned-out and fatigued state you are in, and you are fed up with being tired, ready to reclaim your lost youthful vitality and be successful in all areas of your life, and willing to invest in yourself. Sue will be in contact with you for a fifty-minute complimentary strategy session.

Made in the USA
Middletown, DE
31 July 2016